Occupational therapy
in the community

Occupational therapy in the community

edited by

Eileen E. Bumphrey

Woodhead-Faulkner · Cambridge

Published by Woodhead-Faulkner Ltd
Fitzwiliam House, 32 Trumpington Street, Cambridge CB2 1QY,
England and 27 South Main Street, Wolfeboro, New Hampshire,
03894-2069, USA

First published 1987

British Library Cataloguing in Publication Data
Occupational therapy in the community.
1. Occupational therapy
I. Bumphrey, Eileen E.
615.8'5152   RM735

ISBN 0-85941-329-2
ISBN 0-85941-340-3 Pbk

Library of Congress Cataloging in Publication Data
Occupational therapy in the community.

Includes index.
1. Occupational therapy.   2. Community health
services.   I. Bumphrey, Eileen E.
RM735.035   1986   615.8'5152   86-22429
ISBN 0-85941-329-2
ISBN 0-85941-340-3 (pbk.)

Photo. 8 and Figs 19 and 20 have been reproduced from
Nursing the Aged, edited by Pat Young (Woodhead-Faulkner Ltd)

Designed by Geoff Green
Typeset by Wyvern Typesetting Ltd, Bristol
Printed in Great Britain by
St Edmundsbury Press, Bury St Edmunds, Suffolk

Dedicated to –
Those we seek to serve

Contents

Preface

When approached about a book on 'Occupational Therapy in the Community' two questions were put to me – whether or not one was necessary, and whether I would be prepared to be responsible for it. To the former question I responded in the affirmative, being very aware of the needs of disabled people in the community following current health trends, and the responsibility of occupational therapists towards them. To the latter question, however, it was a very negative reply!

After some thought – and persuasion – however, I realised that no single occupational therapist would be able to undertake such a task and do it justice, as no one therapist would be expert and up to date in all fields of care. Thus, an edited version was born. To this concept I responded as I am very involved with the establishment of community care groups in Norfolk and the needs of the community occupational therapist in these.

If disabled and elderly people are to become members of the community and not relegated to an institutional life, the health and social services, together with volunteers, have to step in to support them at home and to provide them with the assistance to enable them to maintain dignity and comfort. The provision of such services by teams of various professionals, of which occupational therapy is a part, has become a growth area over the past few years, and indeed is continuing to grow, with many initiatives being tried. Thus all professional groups are needing extra help in order to undertake their responsibilities effectively. This book is therefore aimed to help provide part of that required help.

The family, of course, is the primary support for all those we are asked to help and it is essential that they too are cared for. Where there is no family, or they are unable to cope with the extra needs of their disabled member, extra support is necessary to facilitate independence. For those well motivated, little call will be made on the professional services; however, the majority of disabled people will need the services of an occupational therapist to help them over hurdles from time to time. Throughout this book the emphasis has been on the therapist working *with* the disabled person to achieve what he or she wants to do and encouraging a positive approach to assessment, management and treatment programmes.

Many definitions have been given to 'rehabilitation', but within the context of this book it has been kept to the following – 'to restore to privileges' and 'to restore to effectiveness by training'. Rehabilitation therefore is a process in which the disabled and handicapped person is *the* key figure and the occupational therapist's input is seen as one of the many catalysts or facilitators who enables him or her to achieve these. It is a process of solving problems. This does not imply that solutions can be found to all the problems, but it forms a framework for thinking – the 'problem-solving sequence'.

The contributors to this book were invited because of their clinical skills; as experts in their own particular field of care. Their contributions are not intended to be comprehensive, as each felt the need to write a book of their own on their particular subject! However, with the constraints imposed, they have hopefully all achieved to convey to the reader the essence of the aims of treatment and support for their specific disability group and will be of help to their colleagues working in similar situations, especially those who are new to the work of community care. The last contributor is a severely handicapped person representing those we seek to serve. It is those like Phyll who need the skills of the occupational therapist to encourage them to persevere to the ultimate. It seemed fitting, therefore, to invite one of those so handicapped to participate – maybe the last in the sequence of chapters in this book, but certainly not least. I am most indebted to them all for their willingness to participate and the enthusiasm with which they did it.

I am very grateful to Dr Monnica Stewart for agreeing to pick up her pen again to write the introductory chapter for this book. Her approach to health care has been an inspiration to many of us throughout the years and I know will continue to do so. I am also grateful to all those who have encouraged me throughout this venture and have given valuable criticisms and suggestions. My thanks, too, go to my secretary, Christine Richmond, who has admirably coped with the extra work – and the unexpected! – and helped in so many ways; and to my husband without whose incredible patience and support this book would never have materialised.

This book then, is an *introduction* to occupational therapy in the community and hopefully it will inspire many to explore further so that those we seek to serve will achieve their desired goals.

Eileen E. Bumphrey
Norwich 1987

The contributors

Susan Baddeley   Joined the staff at the Norfolk and Norwich Hospital in 1975 after previous experiences gained in London and is currently the Head of Department. Susan has worked in a variety of fields within the physical setting and her current area of work and main interest is with neurological conditions.

Eileen E. Bumphrey   Experience in occupational therapy has been wide, including work in psychiatry, general medicine and orthopaedics, and with severely disabled people, both within hospital and community settings. After a period abroad, in India, and as WHO Consultant in occupational therapy in Taiwan, she returned to Great Britain to undertake research work in Oxford. Eileen has been involved with the development and management of Occupational Therapy services both in Oxford and Norfolk for the past 16 years and is currently District Occupational Therapist in the Norwich Health Authority.

Chia Swee Hong   Gained experience with the mentally handicapped at Chase Farm Village. Currently he works at schools and homes for children and adolescents with special needs in Norwich. He is particularly interested in the development of occupational therapy for people with a mental handicap and has recently completed a post-graduate study in 'Severe Handicap'.

Elizabeth Cracknell   Has had many years practising as a clinical occupational therapist as well as a teaching member of the profession. Currently she is Director of Training at the School of Occupational Therapy, St Andrew's Hospital, Northampton. Elizabeth is trained in counselling and groupwork and applies these skills in her teaching of psychology.

Valerie Dudman   After qualifying as an occupational therapist experience was gained in the Spinal Injuries Unit at Stoke Mandeville Hospital and the Churchill Hospital, Oxford. Valerie has been in her current post of community occupational therapist in Oxford for the past seven years.

Anne Dummett   Qualified as an occupational therapist in 1966 and worked in a number of clinical situations in London and Oxford before going abroad. In Australia she used her previous experience at the Brompton Hospital to devise an occupational therapy programme for chest patients. After a professional break, during which time she explored the intricacies of interior design and financial investment, Anne returned to the Whittington Hospital in London where she developed an interest in the elderly person. She initiated the National Special Interest Group for the elderly and helped pioneer the EDURP Advanced Course for Remedial Therapists in the Care of the Elderly.

Sheila Eden

Experience in working amongst different ethnic groups has been gained whilst working in Tower Hamlets Health District, situated in London's East End, for several years. This area has people of African, Asian, Chinese, Mediterranean and West Indian extraction all bringing together their own culture and subculture to this part of London. Direct contact on a client and professional basis has been gained since 1984 in her present post as the Head Occupational Therapist of the community Health Service.

Lesley Ford

After qualifying as an occupational therapist, Lesley worked in acute psychiatry in Banstead Hospital. Whilst raising a family and travelling with her army husband, she worked in several overseas situations including a spastics school in Singapore and in Kenya. Subsequent family moves led to five years with the social services department in Norfolk before transferring to the Norwich Health Authority to develop psychiatric occupational therapy in the community. Her current position is a new appointment at Maidstone to help establish community services in Kent.

Roger Hadingham

Is responsible for the management of a team of twenty-four social workers covering fifteen hospitals in the Norwich Health District. He has taken a special interest in services for disabled people and is a member of a project team which focuses on the development of local resource initiatives.

Judith Harle

Trained as a nurse at Guy's Hospital, London, followed by midwifery and health visitor training. Following several years as a health visitor, she became a hospital liaison visitor. Both of these posts stimulated an interest in promoting continence which led directly to her present position of continence adviser.

Jean Maclean   Qualified in occupational therapy in 1974. She has held various posts of Edenhall Hospital specialising in the treatment of spinal injuries, and in the community in Livingston New Town. After completing a teacher training course in Glasgow, she joined the staff of the Department of Occupational Therapy at Queen Margaret College, Edinburgh in 1980.

Ann Moy   Began her career as an occupational therapist in 1966 and spent nine years gaining experience in the treatment of physical conditions. In 1975 her interest in design of equipment for the disabled resulted in her appointment as research occupational therapist for the new 'Aids Assessment Programme' sponsored by the DHSS. She has subsequently undertaken several evaluative studies.

Jane R. Page   Has worked in the Norwich area for the past eleven years and has held a variety of positions including work with children, the younger disabled and a continuing care unit. Jane was responsible for setting up the community physiotherapy service for North Norfolk and has worked in this field for four years. In 1984 she completed the Educational Development Unit for the Remedial Professions' Course on the care of the elderly.

Sheila Parsons   For the past seven years Sheila has been the head occupational therapist in a hospital consisting of the younger disabled unit and hospice. Previous experience included neurology and oncology in the district general hospital. For ten years she worked for the local muscular dystrophy group.

Dawn Patterson

Following qualification as an occupational therapist, Dawn gained experience in psychiatry where she became involved in developing a group home scheme for long-stay patients in hospital. Experience in an assessment unit for mentally ill people followed prior to her taking up her current position as a senior community occupational therapist in Lambeth Community Assessment and Treatment Team.

Jill Riley

Before training as an occupational therapist, Jill worked for a short time with mentally and physically handicapped children in Austria. Since qualification she worked at the Newcomen Child Development Centre, Guy's Hospital, London and for one year at a school for physically handicapped children in Essex. Currently she is the head occupational therapist for paediatrics, Jenny Lind Unit, Norwich.

Hilary Shaw

Following her qualification as an occupational therapist experience was gained in acute psychiatry before moving into a community post with the Grampian Regional Council, Aberdeen. Her current position is community occupational therapist with Oxfordshire Health Authority with particular responsibility for the City of Oxford.

Monnica Stewart

During 25 years in geriatric medicine, Dr Stewart helped pioneer multi-disciplinary team-work through films such as *New Beginnings* and *Stroke/Counterstroke* and a book, *My Brother's Keeper?* She contributed to the Open University course, Physically Handicapped Person in the Community. From 1973, she has been a strong campaigner for the provision of comprehensive community support for old people in need. In 1979 she worked in community health in the Newham Health District and she is now Principal Medical Officer (Adult Health) for the Basingstoke and North Hampshire Health Authority.

Phyllis Western   Contracted poliomyelitis at the age of fifteen years which resulted in her becoming severely disabled. Despite this she has led a very full life. A period at the Mary Marlborough Lodge, Oxford, helped her towards a better quality of life. After periods in two residential homes, she now lives at home, supported by two community services volunteers. Phyllis is an active member of the local PHAB Club and participates in many local activities and sports. She has sailed around the Isle of Wight and has travelled abroad.

Chapter 1

Introduction

DR MONNICA C. STEWART
Principal Medical Officer (Adult Health)
Basingstoke and North Hampshire Health Authority

Community care can have a multitude of meanings to a myriad of people. It is an imprecise term, in some contexts being akin to a dirty word, in others indicating the best way of doing things. It would be worth considering how this polarisation may have come about and whether there is a way of eliminating some of the gloomier thoughts and highlighting the positive aspects of the subject.

The medical model has been much used as the basis for all the disciplines concerned, loosely referred to as the greater medical profession, and if one thinks about the conventional training of doctors, especially that of the general practitioner, the lynchpin doctor of community care, then perhaps some of the strengths and weaknesses of the system become easier to understand.

One of the more cheering events of recent years in the National Health Service has been the introduction of vocational training for general practice. The necessity for doctors to spend specific periods in preparatory training, not only in general practice itself supervised by selected and experienced trainers, but also in relevant hospital specialities, such as geriatric medicine, psychiatry, obstetrics, paediatrics or accident and emergency, to name but a few, makes for a much more rounded practitioner. As these six-month appointments are arranged by trainees rotating through different clinical specialities, it means that lateral mobility is beginning to permeate the service.

The inception of the NHS in 1948 unexpectedly tipped the delicate balance of relationship between hospital consultant specialist –

mainly teaching-hospital based – and the family doctor who had beds at his disposal either in local voluntary hospitals or private nursing homes. He usually had, too, some specialist expertise himself in a chosen area of work. Pre-NHS, the teaching hospital was the centre for more esoteric consultant opinion; simpler problems were dealt with locally by fellow general practitioners who had made a particular study (of obstetrics, surgery, anaesthetics, for example) their own speciality.

After 1948 there followed a very positive drive to spread excellence to every part of the country, so that every health district, whether it had a medical school or not, would have the same access to expert specialist help when needed, locally available, and the patient would not need to travel to centres of learning, particularly London, where the greatest concentration of talent was found in twelve great teaching hospitals.

Inevitably, therefore, money was channelled towards the big hospitals and where there were none of adequate size in health districts, plans were made to build them, or bring together smaller and more isolated units to make corporate district general hospitals. At the same time the various colleges of medical specialities began to require that their members achieve measurable standards of excellence by post-graduate training and examination, similar to those of the Royal Colleges of Physicians and Surgeons.

It became less easy for the family doctor to become a specialist as well as being a general practitioner, and without the relevant qualification and formal appointment and grading he would receive no extra remuneration. Gradually the creative tension became apparent between the specialist hospital doctor with considerable sophisticated resources at his command and the 'non-specialist' family doctor with very few resources to call upon. Some of the hospital fraternity began to view the general practitioner as one who had failed to become a specialist and for whom there was no other opening but to descend into general practice and to end his days merely treating the dross of health problems, whilst the more exciting, glamorous work was dealt with by the 'real' doctors, the hospital-based 'giants'. These giants were also the gatekeepers for that much-prized and valuable commodity, the hospital bed, for private nursing homes and small community-based voluntary hospitals had by and large been phased out in the name of clinical excellence and economy.

The recent regrowth of private hospitals, nursing homes and private insurance schemes, the resurrection of community hospitals and the realisation that big is neither beautiful nor very comfortable, has brought about a change of some consequence in the creative tensions in the medical hierarchy. The Royal College of General Practitioners' increasingly firm grasp on the training of their members is not only gaining greater respect for the qualifiers but the lateral mobility of trainees mentioned earlier is bringing change into the walled-off hospital communities previously blissfully unaware of what was really going on in that nebulous entity – *the community*: the place where people live and cope with disability, ill-health and handicap 99.5% of the time, aided and abetted (or not as the case may be) by their families, friends, neighbours, primary health care teams, social services and voluntary organisations.

This being the case a future historian would be forgiven for asking why the monolithic Department of Health and Social Security, with all its resources and power, had not concentrated more effort into building up properly structured support services for the 99.5% of the population in the place where it was most needed – that is, in their own homes, or in other words, *the community*.

It would be easy to attribute any happening to only one cause, but there does appear to be a key element in the construction of this top-heavy edifice which may indeed be at least one of the root causes if not the main one. This is the fact that all the major disciplines comprising the greater medical profession, doctors, nurses, physiotherapists, occupational therapists, radiologists, dentists and so on, receive the major part of their training in a hospital setting. At the most impressionable time the imprint of the hospital hierarchy is stamped upon them and remains indelibly fixed, even if subconsciously, for life. The hospital is the apex of medical life and the workers are the 'cream'. This impression is inevitably passed on to the media and the general public. Hence the easy capitulation of the majority, that it is right to be born and die in hospital, rather than in one's own home; though the latter would, common sense and instinct suggest, be the best possible place for such natural and inevitable events to occur. Usually, people function best and most comfortably in the security of a known environment. Therefore, when one is in a negative state of health one needs all the reinforcement of normality and familiarity to help redress the balance. Any move into unfamiliar territory with unknown personnel to minister to one requires profound thought before such a radical upheaval is embarked upon.

A trainee in general practice presented to the weekly tutorial group a situation which still remained clear in his mind many years later. It went like this. During a Friday afternoon's surgery he was called out to deal with a home emergency. A 50-year-old woman returned home a few days previously, having had an operation (a hysterectomy) in the local district hospital. It was clear to the doctor that she was obstructing and needed urgent re-admission for further surgery of a life-saving nature. This was straightforward: a telephone call to the surgical firm at the hospital who immediately accepted her. The real problem, however, was the patient's 85-year-old mother who was almost blind and deaf, with whom the patient shared a house. Another daughter, who had organised her life and family to come and look after her mother whilst her sister was in hospital, had gone home and could not be brought back in time for this emergency. What was the trainee GP to do? He reported to his trainer that he had had to suspend his other activities in order to deal with this crisis. The trainer wisely held his counsel but stayed available when he heard the course the trainee was proposing, which was a request to the social services to take over the care of the old lady. Discussions between the trainee, the duty officer and the social worker for the deaf and the social worker for the blind brought no solution as the lady was not a client known to them. No vacancy existed in the residential home and there were no emergency cover services to spare to go into the home to help. The next move was to contact the consultant in geriatric medicine for a hospital bed to cover the crisis period. After endless telephoning to hospital departments – eventually a consultant was found who was certainly willing to help – but there was no empty bed to be found.

The situation looked impossible. The time was now 5 pm. The trainer then offered the telephone number of the organiser of the local church community help group who willingly helped by arranging a rota of members to go in and help the old lady in her own home, where she was able to remain amongst familiar surroundings and known hazards, able to follow her usual routine without the extra help she would have needed in a strange territory.

The best possible solution was found to enable this person to continue living as independently as possible. Someone almost blind and deaf is severely handicapped in strange surroundings and amongst strangers; in addition, her obvious great age would inevitably colour the attitudes of new carers and the odds are that this very vulnerable woman would have been reduced to a totally dependent (even incontinent if she could not work out the geography or special routines of the institution) 'geriatric', with all the connotations that this word has come to have. In hospital her needs would have ranked low as she had no illness; in a residential home with low staffing levels and shortage of trained personnel she would also have been at grave risk of being a name and room number and little else. It is alarming to think how close she came to losing dignity and independence.

This whole situation was viewed by the assembled tutorial group of doctors as yet another instance of the total incompetence of the statutory authorities to cope with a simple crisis properly and how yet again voluntary services had had to bail them out – such is the insidious nature of professional training which causes the mind to run along well travelled grooves in times of crisis. There must be an institutional solution to the problem. Yet the ordinary human being and non-professional would see that in this case the right optimal solution had been found. 'Surely prison is an exclamation point and every asylum is the question mark in the sentences of civilisation', as the sage S. W. Duffield commented.

This may seem a long-winded way of introducing a book on occupational therapy in the community but it is relevant as will be seen. Occupational therapy training has been one of the sanest disciplines, firmly keeping in sight the need to treat both mind and body as a whole, and ensuring that students get as varied a clinical experience as possible in the time available. As a result the trained therapist has had the experience of at least four quite disparate clinical settings, meeting many styles of management, both clinical and administrative; whereas some of the students of other disciplines may never have to move away from their own health district, let alone hospital, throughout their training.

The origins of occupational therapy, as mentioned in the next chapter, were very much home and community based and the 1970 Chronically Sick and Disabled Persons Act gave the needed impetus for therapists to move out of the hospital back to the grass roots, largely under the aegis of social service departments. As an intensely skilled and practical profession, the influence they have been able to exert on the attitudes and thinking, both within social service and environmental health departments of local authorities, and also within primary health care teams, has been most marked, where time, opportunity and personality have been able to coincide opportunely.

None the less, as shown in this book, from time to time institutional training may become apparent and jar the susceptibilities of the normal independent adult, giving rise to the question: 'Is that what will happen to me if I have to seek help at some juncture of personal crisis?' These situations can arise purely from therapists working in isolation under stress and without like-minded colleagues available with whom to discuss any ideas.

When circumstances become overwhelming and too much is being asked and expected of one professional and there is no time to breathe, think quietly or discuss with other disciplines, then one is forced back onto known solutions, and traditional ways of coping. There is no time to question whether such answers are appropriate to the specific current dilemma, and institutional answers to society's problems have become accepted by the majority of the population since Victorian times.

There are signs, however, that the climate of opinion is beginning to change. My own came in 1973 after a professional lifetime of trying to make a hospital like home for elderly, disabled patients. A trip to Sweden revealed the fact that even the most sumptuous and well designed environment could never make hospital like home for an elderly person or indeed any age of person. Unless – and the thought is alarming – the previous environment or conditions have been so appalling that an institutional life is a welcome haven.

From 1973 onwards, the inevitable route seemed to be to make the facilities of the hospital available to the sick old person at home. When it became clear that such was the power of the institution over its employees to resist change, working from a community adult health base seemed the only logical progression.

So for this particular community-based health worker, the last years have been magical, almost like coming out of a long dark tunnel into the light. Suddenly finding that people, rather than patients, exist and are alive and well and functioning as members of their community despite the fact that some are dealing with far more formidable disabilities and health problems than some of their peers languishing in a long-stay hospital bed or in a residential home place.

What makes the difference? What makes one person a resident in a young disabled unit (YDU) and another a local authority rate payer, living in a council flat or a privately owned bungalow? Is it the type of disability? Is it the personality? Is it the number of family members available to help? Is it the primary health care team's input? Is it social services provision? Is it the part of the country in which he lives? Or is it purely the amount of personnel available to help? Patently the answer lies in all these aspects, though one thing that is clear and strikes those that know again and again, for every severely disabled or sick person in an institution, there are many more, equally so, coping somehow in their own setting in the community. And if this is so as is undoubtedly the case, why can we not so structure our resources that everyone who *wishes* can be supported in their own chosen setting?

It is said that many people who reside in YDUs and similar institutions have chosen to be there and would be nowhere else. This may have been so initially when the alternative was perhaps between being a total burden on a loving relative or to live alone in unimaginable discomfort and squalor. But times have changed. Peoples' expectations of leading a full life, whatever their physical or mental disability may be, are so much higher, which means that their expectations of professional advisers and helpers are also so much greater. We are being confronted daily by challenge, and all too frequently too many of us are responding to those challenges by forcing the patient into the straitjacket solutions of the traditional past, dredged up from training experiences. When there are too few being called upon to do too much for too many, this will be a foregone conclusion.

How do we get the equation right? So much of it currently depends on post-basic education and this book is very much part of that process. In it, a number of exponents of the gentle art of meeting the supreme challenge of coping bare handed with the health problems of people living in their own homes have shared their experiences with others who may be meeting similar situations or about to do so. This can only be good, with both sides gaining; the writer by taking stock of his practice and underlying philosophy and rationale behind it, the reader by matching it with his own practice and experience, weighing up where to change his methods or to dispute that with which he disagrees, always bearing in mind the infinite capacity of the human mind to resist the introduction of fresh knowledge when it is already overloaded.

Meanwhile, we must continually press that medical education is based primarily on the promotion and maintenance of good health in the community, and secondarily, on the necessary support in times of health crises in the individual person's own choice of setting, or the support of long-term disability or illness. Lastly, only such situations that can only be dealt with in a special place such as hospital or particular type of residential home should be so admitted. If training was based on such a premise and carried out from normal bases of education, with the institutional side forming only a *small* part of a wide spectrum of clinical experience, then we might possibly reach a time when even the professional would be motivated into considering how we could support this person in his or her own home and what resources are necessary to call in to help, rather than, 'How do I get this person into an institution to be looked after and his crisis coped with?'

It is not lack of financial resources that are presently blocking this forward path – rather it is *attitudes*. The money is there but in the hands of those with vested interests and beliefs dedicated to maintaining the *status quo*. The separation of health and social services into differently funded entities started the decline, and subsequent reorganisations of both have done little to right the matter; even the brilliant idea of joint financing has only scratched the surface of joint co-operation and co-ordination. The family practitioner committees becoming free-standing bodies continues the tripartite situation; whilst voluntary bodies, the fourth pillar of structured community care, act in a purposeful working partnership rather than as a stopgap measure. They are funded from many different sources, from central government to local fund raising, that it is impossible to start, particularly when so many exponents have no real faith that this is the right thing to do, because their basic training has conditioned them against it. And nowhere as yet in the whole country is there a total fully fledged structured and functioning community care service (available by a telephone call for anyone who suddenly requires it) to act as a model for all to see and gain faith that it can be done.

Recently (1985) The Prince of Wales' Advisory Group on Disability convened a working party with representatives from over thirty voluntary organisations plus some individuals from the statutory side. The task was to formulate guidelines for those planning services for people with severe disabilities. Interestingly, though it had been the original intention only to look at the age group 16–64, when *Living Options*[1] was eventually published, it was clear that age was not the relevant component, disability was, and that the starting point in any consideration must be to:

1. *Recognise* that those who are affected by disability are people first and disabled second and have individual attitudes, likes, aspirations, fears and abilities.
2. *Understand* that although there may be special areas of need, people with disabilities wish to have the opportunity to live in the same way as other people.

If one takes these two statements together and applies them to all the sections of this book, be it the chapter on mental handicap, mental illness, severe disability, terminal illness, elderly people, or disabled children, then one can use them as a sort of litmus paper.

For an occupational therapist to function at such an individual level all the time may seem to be an exhausting way of working initially, but it is the only effective way of achieving one's goals, and the compensations that accrue are tremendously rewarding.

Having become really person-at-home orientated and determined to help that person achieve whatever autonomy of daily living he or she is striving for, we have to guard against our training once more when the patient asks for help to get outside four walls and do something. The gradual move over recent years from a hospital patient lying passively in bed has followed a predictable path, to the patient sitting in a chair by the bed, to a table in the middle of the ward, to a day room off the ward. From day room to out-patient department, then to day hospital, exchanging bed in ward to bed at home en route. From the day hospital the moves progress to day centres, social centres, work rooms, luncheon clubs, sheltered complexes of one type or another with centralised transport and facilities being provided for specific ages or groups of disabilities. Leisure, work, education and housing and counselling all need the same mode of application. One 15-year-old may not have the same interests as another 15-year-old, just as one 90-year-old does not necessarily have the same affinity with another nonagenarian. On the other hand, a 15-year-old and a 90-year-old both ardent philatelists or cellists might have a great deal in common, even though one might have spina bifida and the other be an amputee.

As we move out of institutional-building thinking, we have to beware of still thinking institutionally about ways of providing activities for large numbers of people, seemingly in need of professional help. It is amazingly easy to set up community institutions in order to rationalise scarce expertise or provide transport to get immobile people out of the house. In one's eagerness to provide answers, it is possible to overlook all the natural everyday resources that are available to the ordinary citizen, both for education and leisure and recreation. It may take longer to set up individual programmes based on existing facilities, but in the long run a more satisfied person will be the result, who is less likely, therefore, to keep reappearing on one's caseload.

We listen and read daily about the 3 million or more unemployed people in the land, but there are also many thousands of people, some say 2.5 million, who are in need of the sort of help that requires another human being, or several human beings in rotation. To solve both problems costs money. Yet if there was universal conviction and faith that institutional care could be slimmed down, the money realised from institutional maintenance would more than pay for the needed human hands and there would be very few remaining institutional problems.

Dr Geoffrey Spencer demonstrated this many years ago on Phipps Ward at the South Western Hospital. Given two willing, though untrained, care attendants working in rotation, a person in a tank respirator could live alone in the community, provided there were the expert back-up facilities needed. Phyllis Western, writer of Chapter 18 is one such person. It is amazing how long it is taking to obtain similar freedom for less heavily dependent people such as para or tetraplegics. The community service volunteers took up the challenge and have been able to show how efficacious the system can be. It can be done. What stops it? The answer must lie within the professional will or lack of it.

So we are back at the beginning again – doctors' training is beginning to get more 'reality orientated'. Students are being encouraged to take their electives abroad preferably in third world countries to see how they cope and how other people live. Medical students are consequently (too slowly, some may think) questioning the relevance of some of their training. The remedial professions too are coming out of hospital hot-houses into polytechnics and universities for their academic education. Occupational therapy has been in the forefront of leaving the sheltered clinical precincts to face the stress and strife of life amongst the social services. Maybe the rest of us will follow suit and, by so doing, help to influence by example the basic training syllabuses.

Meantime this book will help many people in various disciplines not only to understand what occupational therapists are striving and succeeding in doing in the community, but also how the readers may adapt their own custom and practice towards giving much more customised help to the patient/client or person with whom they are in a professional relationship, or who may just be a neighbour or family member.

We are living in a very new era and our working methods must reflect this, not only for those already mentioned but rather as a matter of enlightened self-interest. We shall all of us become old one day, and this is still a disadvantaged condition in our society. It would be heartening to think we might be able to retain our individuality right to the end.

Reference

1. *Living Options* (1985) Guidelines for those planning services for people with severe physical disabilities. The Prince of Wales Advisory Group on Disability. Room 142, 222 Marylebone Road, London NW1 6JJ.

Chapter 2

Providing a service

EILEEN E. BUMPHREY
District Occupational Therapist, Norwich Health Authority

Occupational therapists have been working in a variety of settings within the community for a number of years. In the 1920s voluntary organisations provided craft activities to the homebound, mainly those sufferers of tuberculosis, which became an early form of occupational therapy. These activities were gradually taken over by local authority health departments and between the 1930s and 1970 many legislative changes relating to the disabled and elderly occurred in both health and welfare services which affected the provision of these activities to the homebound. For the welfare services, the guiding principle was to ensure that everyone who was disabled was given the opportunity for sharing in and contributing to the life of the community in which they lived – a principle that should still be adhered to today. On the other hand the NHS Act of 1946/49 was concerned primarily with providing medical treatment and caring for the sick. The occupational therapist could be seen fitting into both of these spheres of care.

After the Second World War, few hospitals offered rehabilitation. Patients sat immobile in hospital beds for several weeks on end and then timidly went home. Fortunately during the past decade this has gradually changed. Patients are now encouraged to rise from their beds as early as possible, follow structured exercises, receive positive rehabilitation and knowledgeable reassurance. In psychiatry, too, patients' treatment programmes have changed with many being successfully treated outside the large psychiatric institutions provided adequate support is given.

In hospital, doctors alone hold clinical responsibility for their patients and it is up to them whether or not they concern themselves beyond the clinical problem presented to them. The patient does not necessarily suffer as the result of this, as the ward sister and other personnel mobilise the services that he or she may need on discharge. However, it is sometimes questionable whether some patients benefit at all from certain hospital-centred treatment. For example, the travel involved to and from hospital for out-patient treatment often negates the actual treatment given because of the inordinate distances involved and time taken in travelling.

On the other hand, dependent patients at home must rely on the perception and energy of their GPs towards the identification of their non-clinical needs and the mobilisation of resources necessary to meet these when the task in question is beyond the capacity of the family. Many essential aspects of the patients' treatment and care also lie outside the fields of both clinical medicine and nursing. These are often more easily recognised within the hospital setting where paramedicals and social workers are involved as a team in the total care, whereas the majority of GPs depend on their attached nurses and health visitors to identify and initiate the services required.

Traditionally the occupational therapist became hospital based until the introduction of the Chronically Sick and Disabled Persons Act in 1970. This Act prompted the employment of many more occupational therapists within the local authority social service departments. They were also given the wider remit of working with disabled people in the community mainly within their own homes. Consequently, in most areas throughout the country, a dual service has arisen with health service personnel being responsible for hospital referrals with those from the community being the responsibility of the social service therapists. The two services present two philosophies and it is the marrying of these two that brings about a successful and supportive service to those who need it most.

Possibilities of providing a unified health and social service support for the home-bound disabled person faded in the early 1970s when the NHS Reorganisation Act (1973) transferred the responsibility for the social support of the sick from the health authorities to the newly formed Local Authority Social Services Departments (LASS). The question still remains: Where does 'clinical medical need' end and 'social care' begin? Because of the constant problem of 'bed blockage', hospital doctors began to take more interest in community-based patient care than before, especially as many of their patients needed basic support rather than skilled nursing care. Joint planning teams, involving hospital, community health and LASS personnel, were set up to provide a forum for the exchange of views and ideas, but unfortunately they had little influence on determining policy decisions. They have subsequently been disbanded.

The emphasis is now on *care in the community*. This embraces two facts – the transfer of patients into 'the community' and the subsequent closure of hospitals (mental illness and mental handicap in particular) and patients remaining in their own home where help and treatment is given so as to prevent hospital admission – 'community care'. These two aspects pose many problems for all agencies concerned as each have their own specific areas of responsibility towards disabled, handicapped and elderly people as shown in Fig. 1. All these agencies have differing bureaucratic systems as well. For example:

1.   Funding: from taxes, rates, or fund raising.
2.   Political bias: especially between central and local government.
3.   Policies: do NHS and social service policies agree? Do local and central government policies agree?
4.   Legislative responsibilities.
5.   Geographical boundaries: NHS and social service boundaries are not always coterminous.
6.   Names: patients, clients or consumer?

Somewhere amongst it all is the poor confused handicapped person needing help – but where to go? The consumer needs to know of the existing statutory legislation and to know where help can be gained.

With these recent changes many hospital-based therapists now find themselves becoming increasingly involved in pre-discharge home assessments and other community-based activities. Around the country many variations on a theme are seen where rehabilitation is taking place outside the institutional environment and in more realistic situations for the patient – for example, at health centres, schools and group homes. Many of these will be discussed in the following chapters.

Occupational therapy is one of many disciplines and services available to disabled and handicapped people today. Their skills are becoming recognised more and more in facilitating the disabled and

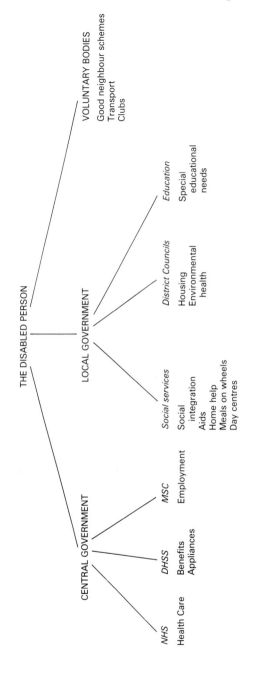

Fig. 1 The provision of care in the community.

the elderly person to achieve maximum independence and to become as fully integrated as possible within the community in which they live. Many of these people may never need hospital admission and therefore will not receive the help they need unless it be provided in the community.

Fortunately today it is not seen as the prerogative of either the NHS or the LASS to provide a community-based service – both have something to contribute in conjunction with other care staff.

Occupational therapy within social service departments

Occupational therapists employed by local authorities work within a variety of structures and under a number of different titles – e.g. rehabilitation adviser/officer or a daily living adviser. They are usually based in the local offices of social services departments working within or alongside the social work team with management arrangements varying enormously around the country. In many instances they are the only occupational therapist within the social work team and are entirely responsible for providing an occupational therapy service to disabled people within the teams' catchment area. Some therefore work in isolation, whereas others may have the professional support and supervision of a senior occupational therapist, with others having the line management to a head occupational therapist.

Occupational therapists are frequently the only group of staff within a social service department who have a medically orientated training. They are therefore often called upon to give advice and help with matters relating to those with physical handicap. With an ever increasing number of these referrals to social service departments, the help of the occupational therapist is being sort with increasing frequency, especially for help with the elderly populace. Unfortunately, however, in some parts of the country their skills are not always recognised when the needs of those with mental illness and mental handicap are being considered, as not all social services managers appreciate the extent of training that occupational therapists receive and their expertise.

Much of the social service occupational therapist's work centres around the provision of aids, and the adaptation of homes. The range of available aids is extensive and continually expanding – some of which are incredibly expensive whereas others are very reasonable. The occupational therapist is therefore expected to know details of all these aids by their clients and others, and to be an expert in this field. Consequently, with the rapidly increasing recognition of the occupational therapist's role and the subsequent rise in the number of referrals, there is the danger that the therapist just becomes the provider of an aid, rather than having the time to fulfil the full role as a therapist by considering alternative means of achieving the task in question which may be far more beneficial, and appropriate, for the client. Also, there is the additional danger that other aspects of care that may be required by the disabled person and his family may be overlooked.

Within any social service department there will be a large amount of administration for the occupational therapist to undertake, although this will vary from authority to authority. Such records as the registration of those with handicaps as required by grant applications and statistical returns are all needed and the occupational therapist will be required to help with these tasks.

Most departments now employ their own technicians and/or aids fitters to make individual aids and to carry out minor adaptations to homes – such as the fixing of hand rails and banisters. They usually work under the supervision of the occupational therapist.

Technical officers and architects in housing and other local authority departments look to the occupational therapist for advice on design of necessary home modifications and adaptations to meet individual requirements. Housing and environmental health departments will frequently only authorise expenditure after an occupational therapy assessment. In addition, their advice may be requested on the design of residential units, group homes and public buildings.

In some areas around the country, the social services occupational therapists are becoming increasingly involved with the development of day and residential care of the mentally ill, rehabilitation programmes for the mentally handicapped, and training programmes for the blind. Overlap with the NHS services will be inevitable especially where there are long established hospital practices. Close liaison between the two services therefore needs to be forged.

Occupational therapy in the NHS

In a few instances, occupational therapists employed by the NHS are seconded to the social services department and as such work in similar ways to those described above. Others work from health authority premises acting as advisers to the social services officers, whereas others provide a full therapeutic service to the community.

It is only in the past decade or so that district therapy services have been empowered by the DHSS to be involved with the needs of the community. Hence, hospital-based occupational therapists have become more involved in home assessments, review procedures and in some cases accept out-patient referrals from general practitioners. However, they too are seldom adequately staffed and equipped to provide all the necessary treatment for patients at home, and in most instances they hold no budgets for the provision of aids and adaptations to homes and therefore need to liaise with their social service colleagues.

Many other disciplines employed by the NHS are also working outside of the hospital environs such as physiotherapists, speech therapists, dietitians and clinical psychologists – too often independent of each other. To the patient they are all 'from the welfare' or 'from the hospital'. Little matters to them just what label they wear (Fig. 2).

The benefits of a strong *primary health care service* lead to the detection of illness, swift treatment to prevent deterioration and

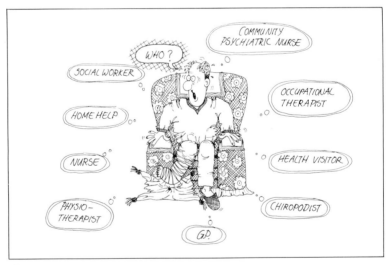

Fig. 2

deformity, and to the care of people within their own homes where the family and neighbours can be supported in their task. Health and local authorities have a statutory duty to co-operate to 'secure and advance the health and welfare' of the population (NHS Act 1977) and therefore it is the duty of the managers of the local occupational therapy services to organise an integrated service.

In many respects, sections of society have come to depend on the health service and the social services more than is necessary for their own good. It is well known that some patients will play one service off against the other. It is therefore essential that both health service and social service occupational therapists work closely together and present a united front.

Planning a community occupational therapy service

No one pattern of management emerges, and this is right. Health authority and social services departments serve districts of differing geographical areas and populations, and the personnel in them plan and experiment with differing initiatives to provide the most appropriate service to their community within the guidelines laid down by the DHSS using the resources that are available to them.

Before an equally distributed health care community service is achieved, further changes within both NHS and social service organisations are needed, including the fusing of area/district boundaries. However, this should not deter any occupational thera-pist from working out a local arrangement with colleagues. Any arrangements that are developed will inevitably be influenced by many factors outside their control – for example, the country's economic position, government policies, and a predominantly elderly population. However, there are some factors over which influence can be made, such as the way resources are used.

The Lund principle drawn up by the World Council of Churches states – 'do nothing separately that you can do together'. This principle is equally applicable to occupational therapists working in the community where a dual service exists. How this is achieved will vary and can only do so when sociological, geographical and industrial factors influencing the needs of the populace are con-sidered. If a rigid imposed structure is implemented, the actual needs of disabled and elderly people could well not be fully met. There is no one right way of providing a service and local decisions will need to be made. However, there are some fundamental principles which need to be recognised – such as:

(a)   A willingness by everyone concerned to work together and respect each other's role and position.

(b)   The head occupational therapists of the NHS and LASS services planning and formalising a common policy.

(c)   Where co-operation between the two services does not occur, understanding by all concerned of each other's differences and problems is needed. Often social service departments will extend over more than one health authority district and vice versa. Only by discussing the differences of laid down policies and trying to formulate some basic principles on which to build a service, can an effective and satisfactory one be achieved.

(d)   The regular review of all policies.

(e)   The problems of one service should be the concern of the other, for as the old proverb says – 'a problem shared is a problem halved'. This will give a deeper understanding of the management and political differences between the two authorities.

When planning an integrated community service the following facts need to be known:

1.   The service that is actually required to meet the real needs of all groups of handicapped and disabled personnel.

2.   The Government's policies and priorities.

3.   The resources available by both services.

4.   The profession's priorities and the local specialist skills that may be available.

Service needs

Despite the success of the NHS, which was aimed at providing improved medical care for all, we still have much chronic disease. Amelia Harris estimated in the late 1960s that some 3.25 million people in Britain had chronic disability.[1]

It is well known that the elderly population is rapidly growing largely due to improved general living conditions and enabling young damaged people to survive into old age. Residential homes, whether local authority or privately owned, now cater for the 80- to 90-year age group, with the 'younger geriatrics' being accommodated in sheltered housing schemes or supported in their own homes.

Large institutions for the mentally ill and mentally handicapped are closing following dramatic changes in the management of these groups of patients. The numbers however remain the same, and therefore a sophisticated health care plan is needed to meet their needs within their own environment.

Government policies

It is well known that the groups of people most at risk are the elderly, mentally ill, mentally handicapped, children and the severely physically handicapped. The Government has given priority for the development of services to these groups and stated specific objectives for their care in the community. Whilst it is appreciated that the details of policies will vary for the different groups, the overall aims remain the same – that is, to maintain the person's links with their family and friends, to encourage as normal a lifestyle as possible and to offer support to meet individual and particular needs. For this to be achieved successfully the policies need to be interlinked with those of the hospitals so that there is a continuum of health care.

Emphasis has also been given on preventative medicine which is an area which occupational therapists have until recently played little part but is one in which thought needs to be given.

Resources

These can be numerous. The following are examples:

1. *Facilities.*
(a) Hospitals have departments which can be made available for all staff to use for assessment and treatment as well as a managerial base.
(b) Health centres often have rooms that can be used for group work.
(c) Local authority residential homes sometimes have accommodation that can be used for specific projects.
(d) Church/village halls could well be available for community-based activities such as travelling day hospitals.
(e) Rehabilitation flats where disabled and handicapped people can be assessed for community living.

2.   *Personnel.* The combined establishment of both NHS and
       LASS services supported by other personnel such as volun-
       teers. Availability of voluntary agencies will vary from place
       to place but their help and support to individual families can
       be extremely valuable.
3.   *Budgets.* For equipment, materials and aids; for travel
       (including cars provided for staff use by the employing
       authority, i.e. Crown cars); training, books and other needs.

Models of practice

Numerous models of management for the provision of occupational
therapy could be described but principles can only be discussed here.
Staffing is the most valuable asset that exists and therefore it is
important that the use of staff is considered critically and objectively.
Primarily all therapists working in the community must be *good*
therapists. They are working in isolation where supervision is not
easy and consequently standards of practise may tend to deteriorate.
Regular supervision needs to be built into any management arrangement together with opportunities for further development. A
soundly basic clinical experience within a hospital and clinical
setting is one of the best forms of training and preparation for the
responsibilities of such an isolated post.

It is impossible for those working either in a generic role or with a
wide variety of disabilities to keep up to date with modern medical
technology and developments in medical care. The back-up of a team
of specialist occupational therapists is needed to support them.
These specialists do not necessarily have to be based within the NHS
(e.g. visual impairment and housing), although the majority do need
clinical attachments (see Fig. 3). The role of the specialist occupational therapist is to advise her colleagues in the management needs
of a particular patient. This may mean a visit to the patient's home or
day-centre or the community occupational therapist accompanying
the patient for hospital appointment. The occupational therapist
may also need extra instruction at the specialist unit.

It is the responsibility of district and head occupational therapists
to give their staff the opportunities for job satisfaction and self
development by taking away the drudgery of non-occupational
therapist duties.

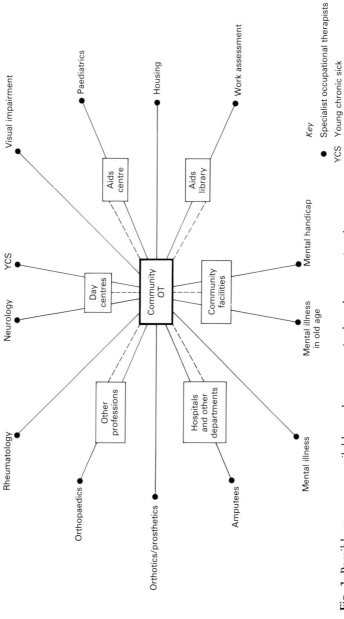

Fig. 3 Possible resources available to the community-based occupational therapist.

Referrals

It is important that there should be as little overlap or duplication of the two services as possible as not only is it a waste of resources, but it can be very detrimental and confusing to the referred person. Consequently some arrangement needs to be made for the acceptance of referrals. For example, with children, it could well make sense for these to be centred with the district handicap team; and likewise those with a mental handicap to the community mental handicap team.

Reporting systems as well as referrals can be standardised and have many advantages. A community care plan system involving nurses, physiotherapists, chiropodists and other colleagues is beneficial and prevents unnecessary overlap and the mystified situation as shown in Fig. 2.

Provision of aids

It is the responsibility of social service departments to provide aids and major equipment for those at home who may need it. However, budgets cannot meet every demand and therefore priorities have to be determined where short-term loans are required – e.g. a raised toilet seat following a total hip replacement could be provided by either the health or social services departments. Long-term loans though are the direct and statutory responsibility of the social services. For items costing over £100 the local authority social services committee's approval is usually required. However, careful assessment of some expensive items needs to take place first before a decision is taken as to whether or not it is correct and meets the person's real needs or is indeed wanted by him. An *aids library* can help in the decision making (see Chapter 11).

One of the major problems in referring the discharged hospital patient to the community occupational therapist is the provision of essential aids and equipment. This can be overcome in a variety of ways – for example,

(a)   Hospital occupational therapy departments hold a stock of social service aids which they issue as necessary.

(b)   Joint aids stores which are centrally situated and available to all occupational therapy staff.

(c)   Red Cross agency supplies aids for immediate issue.

Any system that can be devised to meet the immediate needs of the patient and facilitates early discharge from hospital, or prevent admission to hospital, should be considered by all the local agencies concerned.

Liaison

Occupational therapists are unable to function in isolation and there are numerous agencies with whom liaison is important. Since everyone is required to be registered with a GP, it is obvious that attention must be given to working closely with them as well as their professional colleagues. Other statutory bodies such as housing and education will be discussed in detail in the following chapters. The occupational therapist also needs to be familiar with central and local government departments, charitable and voluntary agencies and the idiosyncrasies of each. Legislation changes with monotonous regularity and all therefore need to be alert to any changes that are made.

Consumer expectations

These are as wide and varied as the people they represent, from accepting any help (appropriate or inappropriate) that is given to them with deep gratitude, to demanding every form of assistance available. Their understanding of what can, or might, be done in treatment or environmental changes are usually based on traditional knowledge, media or neighbourly helpfulness. Disabled people and their families are becoming more active participants in the care process. They ask probing questions, and as they are becoming more informed about their rights, do not give in easily when help is not forthcoming.

The occupational therapist must not expect the handicapped person to conform to the ideals of the professional worker, but with an holistic approach to the needs of the individual, gaining his active participation in solving his own problems, expectations can be effectively met or changed to realistic solutions.

Despite all the complexities of governmental bureaucracy, the links that need to be made with other agencies, and the isolated nature of the work, the community occupational therapist who provides a complete service to the patient or client will gain enormous satisfaction professionally and personally.

By the provision of an adequate occupational therapy service to the community many more people will be helped to remain within their own familiar surroundings, lead a fuller and more interesting life, and hopefully contribute to their own immediate community. The service will also facilitate the early discharge of hospital patients and avoid the humiliation of ending their days in an institution.

Reference

1. Amelia Harris, *Handicapped and Impaired in Great Britain*. London: HMSO, 1971.

Further reading

J. R. Butler and M. S. B. Vaile, *Health and Health Services – an introduction to health care in Britain*, Routledge and Kegan Paul, 1984.
Freda Clarke, *Hospital at Home – the alternative to general hospital admission*, Macmillan, 1984.
Community Care. DHSS, 1981.
Medical Rehabilitation: the pattern for the future. Report of a sub-committee of the Standing Medical Advisory Committee (Mair Report), Edinburgh: HMSO, 1972.

Chapter 3

The occupational therapist in the community

EILEEN E. BUMPHREY
District Occupational Therapist, Norwich Health Authority

It is difficult enough to define occupational therapy in hospital and institutional settings, particularly within the changing face of the Health Service, but in the community it becomes harder as roles between the various professions overlap and merge.

The role of the occupational therapist in the community will vary from place to place, and as the shift of hospital patients into the community continues roles will need to change. Often it will not be easy to adjust to these changes, especially where philosophies are not always compatible and when colleagues do not readily understand the reasoning behind the decisions made.

Role expectations

Role expectations are both perceived by one's supervisor and self-imposed with both being attainable or unattainable, realistic or unrealistic. It is important therefore that both supervisor and therapist are realistic about what should and can be achieved rather than trying only to strive for the ideal and getting frustrated in the process.

The therapist needs to know her limitations, to acknowledge achievable goals and recognise weaknesses. Many believe they are indispensable, giving extra hours to the job, and taking on extra commitments, but in the process becoming overtired, rushing interviews with patients, skipping reassessments, and thus achieving a very mediocre service. All therapists must carefully evaluate their own personal motivations – 'whom do you try to please with your work?' – and regularly review what has been achieved and what has to be left undone. Expectations that are rigid do not lend themselves to alteration and expansion – or even abandonment! Consequently they do not meet the continuing change of the needs of the population. Therefore job expectations need to be agreed, clearly stated, regularly updated and made known to colleagues.

The focus for developing community services must be to provide the right treatment, whether it be assessment, advice, therapy or retraining, for the disabled person in the right place, be it institution, home, work, school, or health centre. In most cases the right treatment can only be accurately prescribed when all services involved take part in determining an agreed programme with the individual concerned and the skills of each used. Consequently the precise role of the occupational therapist will vary from case to case. In many health districts our colleagues, including physiotherapists, are not yet working in the community and consequently the occupational therapist's role may need to include tasks perhaps not normally seen as occupational therapy.

The role of occupational therapy can therefore be extensive, but the primary one remains the same – that is, to develop the optimum level of function and independence in the physical, psychological and social aspects of life, considering age, handicap and environment.

This can be achieved by therapeutic techniques designed to:
1.   Promote and maintain health.
2.   Restore and/or reinforce functional capacities.
3.   Diminish or correct pathology.
4.   Facilitate learning of new skills.
All of these can be successfully carried out in the community by selecting the most appropriate place for each patient where suitable programmes can be expedited.

Specific roles of the occupational therapist within the community

These include:
(a)   The assessment of the individual person's needs and requirements of the family in all aspects of daily living.
(b)   Undertaking planned treatment programmes to achieve maximum independence of the handicapped person or of the family as a unit and prevent disability and dependence.

(c)   Preventing admission to hospital by identifying problems early and promptly and planning treatment within the home or at a nearby day hospital or out-patient department.

(d)   Training home carers, including home helps.

(e)   Evaluating the need for the provision of aids and adaptations to the environment.

(f)   Assessing and advising on employment, leisure, social and recreational activities.

(g)   Continuing treatment programmes begun in hospital in order to effect a return to health or an adjustment to disability.

Other contributions occupational therapists can make are to:

(h)   Special Schools – e.g. therapeutic programmes for individual children and advice to teachers and other staff on specific problems, equipment and architectural needs.

(i)   Handicapped children in mainstream schools – as above.

(j)   Local authority and private residential homes for elderly and handicapped people, advising staff on specific and purposeful activities.

(k)   Day centres – as an adviser and for specific client problems.

(l)   Self help groups – promoting these and advising when necessary.

(m)   Advising on housing projects specifically designed to meet the needs of handicapped people.

(n)   The planning and management of group homes and hostels for mentally ill and mentally handicapped people.

(o)   Other local initiatives that are being explored.

The function and role of the occupational therapist in the community whether employed by the NHS or social services is exactly the same if the real needs of the handicapped person living at home are to be met. Whatever the disability the occupational therapist will need to:

-     Assess the problem, and the person's difficulties in the light of functional abilities and lifestyle required.

-     Undertake treatment programmes in order to achieve the maximum potential.

-     Teach new techniques so as to achieve independence by maximising abilities and minimising handicaps.

-     Provide necessary aids where techniques will not achieve the task required.

- Advise on housing adaptations to overcome environmental problems.
- Develop intellectual stimulation and motivation in order to achieve a quality of life.
- Advise and teach the carers to enable normal interaction and relationships.

All this will need a careful, sensitive and holistic approach to patient care.

The community occupational therapist, especially if undertaking a generic role, needs to have a fund of knowledge if she is to meet all the demands referred to her. This can be overwhelming and can encourage the notion that she is a 'Jack of all trades and master of none'. This must not be the case. There are very special skills needed by community therapists which embrace shrewdness in identifying the person's *real* problem as early as possible and discerning whether help is needed and in what form.

Time will be needed, firstly to gain the person's confidence, to build a rapport and then to give him the time for learning new skills and life patterns as well as for counselling if this is needed. Working with people in their own homes requires more time than that required in other situations. It also requires time for the involvement of the family, as their lives could well be affected by possible changes to lifestyle, and the home environment.

Ethics

The occupational therapist must at all times remember that he or she is a guest in the disabled person's home. It is his private life that is being discussed and as such it must be respected with absolute confidentiality. If the person feels he has no confidence in the therapist in this context little will be achieved. The therapist can in no way impose her ideas; she can only make suggestions. By gentle persuasion and acting as a facilitator she may be able to influence change. However, this change will often necessitate the involvement of each member of the family and in this situation the therapist may need to be a catalyst trying to achieve a compromise from all concerned.

Before embarking on any suggestions for change, especially if it relates to housing adaptations or expenditure of money, it is vital that all the necessary homework is thoroughly undertaken beforehand – for example, it will be important to find out who actually owns the property before any decisions are made as it could be quite likely that a landlord would not agree to the changes suggested.

Where major changes to lifestyles are being recommended the therapist must allow time for all the pro's and con's to be considered in detail; for the family to talk them through; and time to get used to the idea. Also the therapist must not be disappointed if they change their minds and do not accept the suggestions being put forward.

The majority of people referred to occupational therapy readily accept help and advice; however, some, together with their relatives, can be rude and others always complaining. This can make the therapist's task very difficult and unrewarding. Often, however, this is the result of sheer frustration – either with their own disability and the consequent inability to achieve the lifestyle they wish, or disappointment with themselves, or the bureaucracy that they cannot fathom, or indeed it may be due to errors having been made by the occupational therapist or a colleague. Acknowledging mistakes can take the heat out of a situation and will help all to realise that those trying to help are human as well. If, however, major disagreements occur advice will have to be sought and a supervisor consulted. Compatability of personality is not a certainty in professional relationships!

Some disabled people expect the 'professional' entering the home to know everything and this can be daunting! Honesty at all times is essential but it will be important to find out those necessary pieces of information that are unknown as soon as possible.

Confidentiality

With the introduction of tighter legislation relating to protection of personal information, the public are far more aware of this and may react accordingly. Difficulties may arise when attempting to abide by practice relating to confidentiality as well as coping with situations when it is broken. 'Confidence' embraces the idea that there is trust between two people. The nature of the occupational therapist's work often results in her being entrusted with a number of personal confidences – not only those of the person being treated but maybe colleagues as well. Confidences at times are incredibly difficult to keep and this may create many problems for the therapist especially if options have to be sorted out. The therapist must therefore discuss this problem fully and agree what can be divulged and what not and together determine safeguards.

Liaison

The best results in rehabilitation are obtained when all the disciplines concerned work together with the disabled person on a progressive basis towards a common goal. The GP is the first contact responsible for medical care for most of those who are disabled living at home. The Tunbridge Report states that the GP is in a position to initiate the rehabilitation of the patient but he first of all needs to know what is available for him to draw upon. GPs do not necessarily have the time to familiarise themselves with all the resources that are available. On the other hand, home-bound patients rely on their GP to mobilise piecemeal ad hoc services despite the fact that there is no formal requirement for the doctor to concern himself with matters other than the person's clinical needs. Consequently, where the services are not organised in such a way that occupational therapy forms part of the back up team, the occupational therapist needs to make time and effort to get to know the GPs in her area and inform them of their role and the contribution they can make.

Liaison with all the other members of the medical, social and voluntary agencies is also important – for example:

Everyday activities

Washing, dressing	– Community nurses, Bathing attendant
Housework, shopping	– Home helps
Meals	– Meals on wheels
Laundry	– Laundry services
Help with finances	– Social worker Various departments in DHSS
Visit to friends	– Volunteers

Specific needs might include:

Provision of aids	– Occupational therapist, physiotherapist
Wheelchairs	– ALAC DSA
Housing adaptations	– Housing departments
Incontinence	– Health authority or social services

Community treatment programmes might include:

Mobility	– Physiotherapy, chiropody, surgical fitter
Communication	– Speech therapy
Social skills	– Community psychiatric nurse
Pre-work assessment and training course	– Disablement resettlement officer
Assertiveness training	– Psychologist
Relaxation	– Physiotherapist, psychologist, CPN

Working closely together must be the aim of all concerned. Being within a geographical area rather than the tight perimeters of a hospital building, makes efforts to communicate with all colleagues essential and must be regarded as a priority.

Documentation and record keeping is also essential and must be kept up to date. They need to be brief but succinct so that others can act on the occupational therapist's behalf should sickness or other urgent situations warrant this. Messages and cross-referrals must be clear and precise so that they cannot be misconstrued. Whenever possible, common documentation between professions is helpful. A community care plan card on which all concerned with the disabled person can write their comments, placed in a large envelope and put in an obvious position in the home is one way of maintaining links. Into this envelope can be put all the workers' visiting cards, so that the disabled person concerned and his family, as well as colleagues, has the name, address and telephone number of everyone should they wish to contact them.

Another means of informing all disciplines of one's involvement with a particular person is by placing a card in the patient's GP notes – 'the co-operation card'. This need only indicate when an episode is opened and closed and by whom.

Caring for oneself

In the community the experience of isolation and loneliness by virtue of the role and nature of the work is real. The occupational therapist sees herself as continually a 'giver' with little reward. There is little hour-by-hour or even day-by-day support and consequently there is the danger of emotional exhaustion which is not always realised by the person concerned. The therapist has a strong conviction that 'I can cope', 'I can take care of myself', 'I do not need regular support'.

The therapist's self perception of competence and control leads to self-imposed constraints which in turn not only lead to professional limitations but encourages loneliness, failure and lowered self esteem – or sheer arrogance! No one can endlessly give to others as effectively as possible without finding ways of replenishing the emotional resources used. Many therapists also find themselves caught between their own expectations as 'givers' and their need to be cared for when emotional exhaustion occurs or is imminent.

Stress can be prevalent in these situations and therefore the therapist must have an understanding of how to cope with any imposed by management or found within their patients and clients. It is important, therefore, that each therapist knows the stress factors that effect them and work out their own anti-stress strategy – for example,

(a)   Recognise personal physical signs – such as perspiration, heart burn.

(b)   Develop lower level arousal and keep fit activities.

(c)   Change attitudes – by knowing oneself a..d the tolerance level; admitting stress and 'unacceptable feelings'; say 'no' and 'yes' to realities.

(d)   Deal with change – by anticipating changes that may be imposed or are necessary; learn from experiences; discover as many choices as possible to solve problems.

(e)   Build a support network such as a co-counsellor.

Whilst gaining help from friends, family and others, all therapists need a colleague with whom they can relate and share professional problems and concerns. Ideally the concept of co-workers is the best way to help in this – each supporting the other emotionally, sharing experiences, feelings, concerns and problems as well as highlights. A support group which meets on a regular basis facilitates mutual support, enables problem solving discussions and opportunities for sharing experiences. A facilitator may be needed to organise this, but he or she should not be seen as a leader. Professional counselling may be needed from time to time. Such arrangements should be readily available and known to the therapist.

Training

It is essential that all community occupational therapist's keep abreast of current medical practice. Identifying areas of work in which the therapist needs help should be undertaken as early as possible, after an adequate induction period, and a set programme for training established to cover these needs. This should also be ongoing.

All community occupational therapists should complete a recognised first aid course and keep up to date with these procedures. The 'unexpected' can always happen and although this may be very rare it is crucial to know just what to do if faced with such an emergency situation. It is therefore important that the therapist knows how and what to look for in the initial assessment of the situation, and how to react appropriately. First aid is the skilled application of accepted principles of treatment on the occurrence of injury or case of illness, using the facilities or materials available at the time, which often means innovations, to 'preserve life, prevent the condition deteriorating, and promote recovery'.

Accommodation

The environment in which one has to work is important and should be conducive to the type of work that is undertaken. When working in the community, the employing authority often considers that accommodation for the community worker is not necessary because most of the time is spent either in people's homes or in their own car! Access to a telephone is all that is necessary! The need for adequate quiet accommodation, albeit shared with others, is essential. Access to a private room for confidential discussions, telephone conversations and relaxation is also needed.

The actual workspace and the arrangement of furniture can either support or hinder performance. Inadequate space and equipment, such as filing cabinets, leads to clutter, resulting in a poor performance. Cramped and inadequate space leads to frustration. Adequate storage space for aids and equipment is essential and should be accessible to one's base.

Any work situation in which personal energies are drained in order to cope with cramped quarters will reduce one's capacity to achieve the goals set and job satisfaction.

For patient assessment and treatment programmes access to the local hospital occupational therapy department may well be the answer, although the facilities in health centres and other NHS and local authorities properties are possibilities.

Further reading

College of Occupational Therapists, *Resource Book for Community Occupational Therapists*, 1984.

Jane Madders, *Stress and Relaxation*, Martin Dunitz, 1979.

N. MacDonald and M. Doyle, *The Stresses of Work*, Nelson, 1982.

Pamela K. S. Patrick, *Health Care Worker: Burn out – what it is, and what to do about it*, Inquiry Books, 1981.

Chapter 4

The needs of the disabled person in the family and in the community

ROGER HADINGHAM
Area Social Services Officer, Norfolk County Council

'Somehow I expected everything to have changed when I came out of hospital. It was a strange and really quite a frightening experience to leave hospital "different" from when I went in. I expected things to be different because my experience of it had, but in fact it was I who had changed. Hospital was awful – but at least I had a place in it, but at home you are on your own. On leaving hospital I found I was labelled "disabled". I had now entered a very strange and unknown world which was alien, hostile and unloving.'

'Many people still do not realise that inside an immobile body sitting in a wheelchair is a lively mind wanting to express itself and show everyone that he can be independent in his own way, for independence is not only a physical thing – it is a state of mind, telling everyone that "I can do it" – even if it takes me time and I have to ask for a little help. "I'm going to do it!" '

These two quotations from disabled people express some of the frustrations encountered during the 'rites of passage' for the disabled person from being able-bodied through hospitalisation and rehabilitation to independence. There are various stages in this process, each entailing the individual modifying his role and status in order to adapt to the demands being placed upon him. He can only be expected to successfully complete this process if the appropriate 'professionals' in partnership with the individual can identify and meet the needs as they are presented. Some disabled people never get beyond the 'patient' phase, many are never fully rehabilitated, whilst only a minority become fully self-determining. The responsibility for an incomplete journey must be shared between both the individual and the various professional organisations and others whose *raison d'etre* is to assist.

The first phase – hospitalisation

It might appear out of place to discuss the effects of hospitalisation in a chapter devoted to outlining the needs of the disabled person in the community. It is the case, however, that the experience of hospital and the extent to which needs are met in that setting critically influence the ability of those disabled people experiencing such an event to negotiate the rehabilitation phase and reach independence. Furthermore, it is essential for the community-based professional to have an awareness of some of the residual expectations the disabled person carries forward from the time he was hospitalised.

It should also be mentioned that though this section principally focuses on the effects on the disabled person of being hospitalised, many of the points raised are applicable to those who do not commence their disabled lives with a protracted period of hospitalisation. The large group of people born with a physical disability, or those who develop a comparatively slow, progressive condition will also experience some of the characteristics of this induction into a disabled career.

On admission to hospital, the individual is expected to take on the identity of 'patient'. There is a generalised expectation of dependency characterised by an obedience to the rules and norms of behaviour within the institution. The patient surrenders to a large extent his self-determination and accepts the omnipotence of the medical expertise in making more decisions on his behalf. He adopts an expectation that suffering and pain are part of being ill and, to a greater or lesser extent, lives with a measure of diagnostic uncertainty. In short, to be sick is to be defined as in need of help and to co-operate with the 'experts' who are offering this help.

Both because of the power of this pressure to conform to the sick role and the length of time many disabled people spend in hospital at the time of diagnosis, some adopt this role so completely that they are unable to relinquish it. To be disabled becomes synonomous with being 'sick'. The disabled person defers all decision making to his carers and completely lacks the motivation necessary to move onto the rehabilitation phase.

It is essential that hospital staff differentiate between those patients who will probably be permanently disabled and those who are the transitory sick. Those people for whom hospitalisation is a temporary interruption, not necessitating a permanent disruption of their basic lifestyle, are usually able to throw off the mantle of 'sick' and return to their normal role upon discharge from hospital. The patient who is beginning a career as a disabled person is not, however, able to fully return to his pre-admission status or role. He must to a greater or lesser extent adopt a completely new role – a task which is frightening and difficult. To retain the role of 'patient' therefore becomes a seductive alternative.

In addition to the fear of potentially having no place or status within the wider society, the disabled person also has other, psychologically deeper, reasons for not wishing to abandon the umbilical link with the medical services. The hospital staff and particularly the consultant is a source of knowledge in the person's search for a meaning to his newly acquired disability. He has a need to define his condition as a whole, to make sense of his changed world and find a structure within which his disability can fit.

This search for knowledge is a powerful urge within which two distinct stages can be identified. Initially, the person is concerned with locating the cause of the disease or accident which has brought about the disability. He tries to find an answer to the question 'why me?' in terms which fit into the structure of the new world he is forming. Later, he becomes more concerned with the prognosis of his condition. He has to define the parameters in order to facilitate the basic psychological management of the disorder, both in the short and the long term.

The hospital is also a source of hope in the psychological search for an alleviation of the symptoms or even a cure. Discharge from hospital and the subsequent 'loss of interest' by the medical elite is, in the mind of the disabled person, an indication of the permanence of the disability.

Thus the need for effective and repeated communication between doctor, therapist and patient is crucial. In her study of those people discharged during a four-month period from a hospital who were likely to be permanently disabled, Blaxter (1976) found that com-

munication was the one subject about which a great deal of dis-
satisfactions were expressed.[1] Misunderstanding or inadequate
information was identified as arising from one or more of four
distinct courses.

First, there were instances where basic organisational failures in
communication had come about through discrepancies between
different doctors or a failure to explain the results of specific tests or
the effects of particular drugs to the patient. Second, there were
examples of misinterpretation often through the doctor giving either
a too technical or even a too simplistic explanation of a diagnosis or
prognosis. An example of a too simplistic explanation was a doctor
using the term 'nerves' to describe a neurological condition. To the
patient, to suffer with one's 'nerves' was synonymous with having a
psychiatric condition!

A third problem in communication arose where there was a
medical uncertainty about the diagnosis. This obviously presents a
real dilemma for the doctor in deciding the extent to which this
uncertainty should be communicated to the patient. In the short
term, the uncertainty can be interpreted as hope. Whereas, in the
longer term, such uncertainty can further 'disable' the disabled
person through inhibiting the process of re-defining the patient's role
in his family and community.

Finally, Blaxter found some instances where there had been a
conscious decision by the doctors and therapists to maintain a
pretence of uncertainty on the assumption that this stance could, in
certain circumstances, be in the best interest of the patient.

Not only is there a need to feed the patient a continuous flow of
information concerning his condition, there is also a need for each
member of the therapeutic team to reinforce the information
previously given. The anxious patient, given frightening information
in a strange environment, can easily misinterpret the information
given and the opportunity for feedback on the patient's perceptions
of his condition should also be available.

In a real sense, the disabled person needs to be encouraged to
personally and systematically take on the responsibility initially
vested in medical and nursing staff. In order to maximise his
independence once back in the community he needs to be able to
manage his own condition. Obviously, this can only be achieved
with considerable assistance at the relevant crucial stages by the
various professional therapists. Equally essential in this process

however is the access to the basic information about the condition. It is not only in an Orwellian world that information can be equated with power.

The second phase – rehabilitation

Once the acute phase of the hospitalisation process is over, the disabled person should be received into a regime where maximum restoration of independence should be the norm rather than the provision of care. The different models of patient care are detailed in Table 1 and highlight the many differences between the 'classical' model the disabled person is leaving and the 'rehabilitative' model which he ought to be entering at this stage in his career. The 'custodial' model has been included in Table 1 as it represents the alternative career for those disabled people who are unable to cast off the temporary sick role. Such disabled people need not necessarily be habilitated in an institutional setting, and may conform to the main criteria of this dimension even though cared for in the community.

The rehabilitation phase commences whilst the disabled person is still a patient in hospital and continues beyond discharge and his return to the family and the community. As the needs of the disabled person become wider so the range of personnel involved increases.

At this point the prevailing view of the person must pass from the medical to the functional. The passive patient becomes the active participant in the rehabilitation process. The emphasis on the functional problems should however be balanced by an awareness

Table 1 Models of patient care.

Dimension	Classical	Rehabilitation	Custodial
Stated goal	Care	Restoration	Comfort
Assumptions about disease process	Reversible	Mutable	Incurable
Therapy	Central	Supplementary	Sporadic
Sick role	Temporary	Intermittent	Permanent
Patient motivation	Obedience to doctor's orders	Achieve mystery	Obedience to institutions rules
Resulting institutional model	Acute general hospital	Rehabilitation Centre	Total institution

of, and attention to, the assets of the person. Too much emphasis on the functional limitations can psychologically disable the physically disabled person at a time when healthy physical and mental attitudes can become a basis in themselves for alleviating difficulties.

As with the hospitalisation phase, it is essential to encourage the active participation of the person in the planning and execution of the rehabilitation programme. This not only enhances his self respect, but also fosters the important development of initiative and responsibility for his own decisions. This participation should not however be limited to the individual as it is important to acknowledge that he is part of a larger social group in the community. The early involvement of family members, close colleagues and friends is essential at this time.

The significance of the eventual handicap from which the disabled person suffers will be affected by the feelings he has about himself and his situation. Feelings of resentment, inferiority, guilt and loneliness are common features during this phase. The disabled person is also addressing such issues as whether he can still be loved in his family and valued in his workplace and community. Residual feelings of dependency from the acute hospitalisation phase and frustrations at his lack of expertise in mastering his disability can mean inhibition of physical progress by psychological despondency.

Though the need for counselling at this time is important, the emotional well-being of the person can equally well be helped by dealing appropriately with the realities around him rather than 'treating' his feelings in a vacuum.

Thus far the rehabilitation phase has been identified as taking place within the hospital setting. It must, however, bridge the patient's return to the community – a traumatic transition for every disabled person as evidenced by the woman quoted at the start of this chapter. Progress and adaptability within the cloistered setting of the hospital are subjected to a severe test; back in the community a familiar setting can easily be seen as 'alien, absurd and ultimately defeating'.

The common experience of a temporary relapse in the rehabilitation process heightens the person's awareness of his disability and the changes in his social role consequent upon that disability. At a time when there is an often frightening acknowledgement of the need to redefine the place in the family and wider community, it is important that strong links remain with the medical and therapeutic team. If the recently discharged disabled person conceives of having no place and no status in the wider society, he needs to continue to receive 'comfort' from his familiar role in the context of medical care whilst he struggles with this traumatic transition.

The return to the family is not only problematical for the disabled person himself, but it is also a potential source of many difficulties for the other members of the family. This is particularly so if there has been an intimate and loving relationship with the spouse prior to the onset of the disability. The disabled partner is seen as no longer being the same person because of the change in his physical – and maybe intellectual – state. In such circumstances, both partners need to go through a period of mourning for the loss of the original marital relationship as part of the adjustment. The disabled partner often has to learn to accept a fundamental loss of dignity and privacy as the spouse takes on the task of providing a much higher degree of care. The need for the disabled person to relinquish some tasks and the partner to take over can lead to a significant readjustment of their relationship especially if the tasks are as basic as washing, dressing, feeding, supervision of medication and even toiletting. In some instances this takes the form of an adult relationship based on basic equality becoming one essentially of parent and child in order for the marriage to survive.

The able-bodied spouse is further encouraged into the role of parent through being placed in the position of having to take on total responsibility for the home and family. The able-bodied partner takes on the role previously carved out by the disabled person. Thus either the wife has to take on the traditional masculine tasks or the husband is forced to become the 'housewife' within the family – and possibly, at the same time, continue to be the breadwinner.

The necessity of such role reversal can contribute towards enhancing feelings of social isolation and loneliness. Disability impinges on friends and other family members in a variety of ways and reacts back on the disabled individual to reinforce and exacerbate his problems. It is often inevitable that isolation follows from repeated social embarrassment and rejection by old acquaintances.

A disabled child within a family can bring different problems to the family unit as the needs of that child must be met often at the expense of less time being given to the other members. The siblings may react to a lack of attention by displaying behavioural problems, physical problems such as bed wetting, and even penalising their disabled brother or sister. Likewise the disabled child can take advantage of the situation by becoming more demanding to all members of the family – not just the parents.

An elderly grandparent needing help, whether living nearby or within the family home, can also present strains in relationships especially for the mid-generation. The mother trying to care for her young family will find that the pull of caring for her mother or father will bring conflicts of loyalties – loyalty to parent, husband and children. All will demand her attention either collectively or individually. Such intensity of demands cannot help but create strains which could well lead to resentment and rejection of the elderly grandparent.

Access

Once the basic psychological trauma of discharge from hospital and reintegration into the family have hopefully been worked through, then a whole series of more practical needs become evident.

The most basic of these is presented under the umbrella term 'access'. This is most commonly presented in the sense of the need for the disabled person to be ensured of physical access to public places in the community. This has been seen as so basic that it has been enshrined in a number of statutes – most notably in Section Two of the Chronically Sick and Disabled Persons Act 1970. Many local guides are published listing those facilities where there are no architectural barriers inhibiting access and all new designs of public buildings must incorporate this feature. Despite a considerably enhanced awareness of this need, barriers remain. One example is highlighted in one of the recent Spastic Society posters which shows a photograph of a wheelchair bound person gazing in frustration at a public convenience located below street level down a flight of steps. The caption makes the point that this particular toilet is neither 'public' nor 'convenient'!

Important though physical access is, there are several other forms of access which are equally as essential if the disabled person is to be successful in navigating the rehabilitation phase.

Mobility

The breaking up of architectural barriers only gains significance for the disabled person if that person has a sufficient degree of generalised mobility to be in a position to take advantage of improved access to public buildings. The need to maximise mobility is evident on both a micro-level within the disabled person's home and a macro-level within the wider environment. The environment in general is designed by able-bodied people for their like kind. In order for a disabled person to be able to successfully negotiate this world, a multitude of both minor and major adaptations must be made.

The strategies employed to improve mobility in themselves can have considerable psychological significance to both the disabled individual and to the wider public's attitudes towards them. An interesting example is the strategy used to enable independent travel. The light blue three wheeled 'trike' was, until comparatively recently, the standard, obligatory provision in this country. This scheme certainly gave numerous individuals a level of mobility unimagined by the previous generation. However, the freedom it provided was limited. The disabled person had little choice – the 'trike' was the official solution, the specification of which was detailed down to the colour. It was a vehicle designed for a single disabled person and thus failed to acknowledge that most of them do not live alone and like company. Furthermore, the 'trike' was unique to the disabled and bore no resemblance to the mass of other vehicles on the roads. Thus, although the trike scheme did allow greater mobility, it also served to emphasise the difference between disabled people and the rest of society.

Fortunately, this scheme has now been replaced by enhanced financial benefit which allows an individually tailored solution to improved mobility and can be seen as an example of the need a disabled person has for an overall income which covers more than the basic necessities of daily living. It is more expensive to navigate an able-bodied world in which mass-produced, and therefore more economical, resources can not be utilised by the disabled. One of the characteristics of poverty is its effect on limiting activities and options. To experience this when it is coupled with functional limitations can give a disabled person an unbearable dual handicap.

Employment

An adequate income can come from employment. Being in full-time work is also the most common method of fulfilling another need –

the need to have a meaningful way of occupying one's time. The disabled person is often disadvantaged in the degree of access to a full range of opportunities in the fields of both employment and recreation.

Information

Throughout this chapter emphasis has been placed on the significance of basic information to the disabled person. During the hospitalisation phase the need for information is related to details about the diagnosis and prognosis in order to enable the person to manage his condition psychologically. For the disabled person back in the community this need for information is just as crucial but the significance here is on the contribution it makes to enable him to manage his condition practically. During the rehabilitation phase the category of information is that of relating to the range of services – statutory and voluntary, formal and informal – that are designed to help him.

It is still the case that the majority of resources for disabled people are designed and orchestrated by the able-bodied. The need for these becomes more acute as the newly disabled person experiences the erosion of income, wealth and social supports which frequently accompany disability, but often development of a comprehensive information network in order to allow easy access to these resources is neglected.

Many disabled people are thus unaware of the range of potential resources which might be available to them, and it comes as no surprise that the tremendous recent technological advances in the storage and transmission of information has still to make a significant impact on them and those seeking to provide appropriate practical resources to them.

The rehabilitation phase sees the predominence of these professionals whose primary task is to advise and encourage the disabled person to maximise his altered functional abilities. The medical and nursing input diminishes as the focus changes from hospital-based treatment to community-based rehabilitation. The needs of the disabled person are seen not solely as individually based, but as applying to a much more complex system which includes family, friends and the wider community.

There is, however a danger that the relationship between the disabled person and the range of professional 'therapists' can of itself perpetuate dependency. Just as the disabled person must, during the hospitalisation phase, be encouraged to take on some of the responsibilities initially vested in the medical and nursing staff, so must he similarly be encouraged to take some of the responsibilities vested in therapeutic staff during the rehabilitation phase. Rehabilitation is not, after all, an end in itself, but rather it represents the means whereby the disabled person achieves independence.

The third phase – independence

True independence means much more than merely residing in the community. Independence cannot be measured solely by the ability to carry out mundane physical tasks unaided, but more significantly by the range of personal and economic decisions made by the disabled person. The concept of independence must be expanded to include both physical and intellectual achievements – not only the quantity of physical tasks a disabled person can undertake but also the quality of that person's life.

To the rehabilitation personnel who have slowly and systematically assisted in the maximisation of physical resources, the concept of independence means acknowledging the importance to the disabled person of risk-taking. The model of service should thus focus more on planning and creating services with him and less on doing something to the disabled person. Central to this concept is the recognition that the disabled person should no longer be the passive recipient of services. He should be expected to take an active role in designing and managing the basic services he requires.

The basic characteristics of such independence can perhaps best be illuminated through a contrast between two models of community based care – the traditional home help/district nurse model and the attendant care model. The latter model is one whereby the disabled person has responsibility for the recruitment, payment, training and supervision of the 'carer'. As can be seen from Table 2, it is the disabled person, not the provider, who directs the provision of care he needs.

The general concern amongst people with disabilities is that the structures within which services are provided generally foster dependency. This has led to the growth of the Independent Living Movement, first in the United States, but also more recently in this

Table 2 Two models of community-based care.

Home help/district nurse	Attendant
'Professional' definition of needs	Consumer definition of needs
Provider direction	Consumer direction
External supervision	No external supervision
Recruitment by 'agency'	Recruitment by consumer
Payment to carer	Payment to consumer to carer
Accountability to agency	Accountability to consumer
Disabled person has patient role	Disabled person has consumer role

country.[2] This movement represents community-based coalitions of disabled people whose aim is to devise local resources which, with substantial consumer involvement, can provide services to meet the needs of severely disabled people so that their self-determination is increased and dependence on others minimised. In addition to care attendant schemes, such services can range from housing to information on welfare benefits and can even include such activities as peer counselling and advocacy.

The increasing awareness amongst both disabled individuals and some of their formal organisations of the potentially debilitating effects of many of the services ostensibly aimed at fostering independence has led to at least one prominent disabled academic describing the relationship between the disabled and the relevant professional organisations as being at the point of crisis. Though this is perhaps an over-pessimistic view, it should serve to remind us all of the danger of minimising the difficulties we sometimes have in encouraging the person with a disability to meet his most significant need – that of independence.

References

1. M. Blaxter, *The Meaning of Disability*, Heinemann, 1976.
2. Crewe and Zola, *Independent Living for Physically Disabled People*, Jossey-Bass, 1983.

Further reading

J. Campling, *Images of Ourselves*, Routledge and Kegan Paul, 1981.
R. M. Coe, *Sociology of Medicine*, New York: McGraw-Hill, 1970.
D. Locker, *Disability and Disadvantage*, Tavistock Publications, 1983.
D. Thomas, *The Experience of Handicap*, Methuen, 1982.

Chapter 5

Achieving independence

JEAN MACLEAN
Lecturer, Queen Margaret College, Edinburgh

The Shorter Oxford English Dictionary definition of independence
is:

'The condition or quality of being independent; the fact of not
depending on another; exemption from external control or support, individual liberty of thought or action'

and the definition of independent is:

'not depending on the existence or actions of others; not subject
to external control or rule; not dependent on another for support'.

Within these definitions there are degrees of independence. Very few
people are totally independent of all others; to be so would mean
total self-sufficiency, which is possible but unusual in our society.
Most people have some degree of dependence on others. Following
studies with disabled people Dartington, Miller and Gwynne
observed that 'ideology of independence called for greater autonomy
and a capacity for self-fulfilment greater than most "really normal"
people have, while the dependence on others which all of us have and
which those who are physically handicapped have more than most
was defined as a weakness.'[1]

Physical handicap, mental handicap and psychiatric illness all
impose limitations on independence which in turn will affect the
quality of life that can be achieved.

Views of independence

Individual views of independence vary greatly. The newly disabled person looks to the 'best' patient in the ward as a model and perceives that person's level of independence as his initial aim. Slightly longer term disabled people who are hospitalised or in unsuitable accommodation see independence as living in a suitable house and again being part of the family unit. Those longer term disabled people who already live in the family home perceive independence as having a reasonable income, a comfortable home and the freedom to do what they want when they want. It would seem therefore that the nearer a person is to independence in the community the more his perceptions merge with those of non disabled people.

Independence has two distinct stages – short and long term.

Short-term independence

This can be described as the level which can reasonably be reached, in the foreseeable future, during the early stages of treatment or rehabilitation. This often, but not necessarily, occurs within the confines of a hospital. Its achievement depends largely on the person's condition and motivation, and the quality of care available. The amount of care and support required at this stage is usually high.

Initial steps towards independence appear similar for people with congenital and acquired handicap or illness. Initially a protective shield provided by relatives, professionals and other carers direct the individual towards short-term independence. Progress is often fairly rapid at this stage. The patient is encouraged by it and generally responds well to help and support.

A person on leaving hospital is no longer acutely ill but he or she may not be functionally fit. The veneer of short-term care directed at the achievement of short-term independence wears thin. The intensity of support provided gradually decreases and the long-term carers emerge. Input from different professions may be required in helping achieve long-term independence. The rate of progress tends to slow down at this stage.

Long-term independence

This is the optimum level which may be reached in time. It depends on many factors including those found to be important in the achievement of short-term independence. The amount of care required should gradually diminish through time. Setting realistic long-term goals may be very difficult or impossible for an individual whose life has suddenly been affected by an illness or disability. Acceptance of disability or handicap is a necessary prerequisite for the establishment of these goals and many factors will influence the fulfilment of them such as the person's personality, his family, education and financial position.

The disabled individual

The degree of disadvantage through illness or disability is very varied as are individual responses to it. Some people are very passive and accept direction and help without question, whereas others will fight to achieve their own goals, often achieving more than professional carers would have thought possible. It requires great strength of character for disabled persons to supersede pre-set goals. In their effort to do so they may be described as difficult, non-conforming or unrealistic. If they succeed they are admired for their determination but if they fail they are greeted with the attitude of 'I told you so' and discouraged from trying again.

Safilios Rothschild describes a tendency in professionals connected with rehabilitation 'to define the self concepts, goals and inner motivations of disabled people and determine their "real" wishes and potentials.'[2] It is important for health care professionals, including occupational therapists, to consider all aspects of each individual case when setting goals to ensure that they are neither too advanced nor too simple. Above all, goal setting cannot be achieved without the disabled person's positive participation.

The establishment of a self concept which is aimed at maximum independence is important for all disabled people. Our self concept is partly made up of what other people tell us we are and what we can achieve. Thus if a disabled person is smothered and has everything done for him he will accept dependence and may well not attempt tasks he believes are not within his ability. On the other hand, if he is encouraged from an early stage in rehabilitation to be as independent as possible he will accept that as a norm and is much more likely to attempt and achieve a number of tasks.

Most people are motivated to be as independent as possible because of the positive effect this has on self esteem. A few people however have little motivation to achieve independence. They fall into several distinct groups. First, there is a very unfortunate group who feel they are better off in hospital than at home. Most of the people in this group live alone and have few family or social contacts; they see the achievement of independence as living in isolation. These people need to be identified early and given support to return to or remain in a community which helps to give meaning to their lives. Occupational therapists must be aware of all the community resources and facilities which may be available to help them.

The second group whose motivations may be affected, albeit subconsciously, are those who have a compensation claim outstanding following an injury or illness related to negligence or poor working conditions and who are likely to be awarded a higher sum of money if they are more disabled. It is only fair to say that this is by no means the case with every compensation claim, but it is a recognised phenomenon.

The third group are those with a severe progressive disorder, some of whom feel they cannot win in the independence battle because the worsening conditions always defeat them by progressing further to add to their limitations and erode their independence (see Chapter 11).

A further group are those people who are very highly motivated but feel that they had to be selective in tasks to be achieved. If time and effort spent outweigh its advantages, it may be better to compromise and accept help in one area in order to use time and energy for more fulfilling tasks. For example, a child with muscular dystrophy may prefer to use a wheelchair at school so as to conserve his energies for educational activities and play with his friends, rather than expending it all in 'walking' from one classroom to another.

For those people whose motivation is lacking every effort will need to be made to identify the reasons for this so that help can be given to deal with the underlying causes.

The family

One disabled person in the family will affect the other members to a greater or lesser degree and may effectively disadvantage them. Blaxter describes this as 'the disabled family'.[3] Independence for the family is just as important as independence for its disabled member. It is vital that help and support is given and that the family is aware of its availability. All too often professionals deal exclusively with the ill or handicapped person in isolation and the needs of the whole family are not considered – or even identified – until a crisis arises. If people appear to be coping it is often assumed that all is well – this in fact may be far from the truth, for it may be that the family do not know what help is just round the corner. Also, they may not like to ask for help or to admit that they are experiencing difficulties. Awareness on the part of the occupational therapist of potential problems and discussion with the relatives about any difficulties or apprehensions that they may have may well avert a crisis situation developing.

Family attitudes towards a disabled member may well determine the success or failure of attempts to achieve independence (see Chapter 4).

Housing

The type of housing available from area to area is very different. Some towns have a good deal of housing suitable for wheelchairs or for use as group homes – others have very little. The design and location of housing is vitally important in achieving independence. A house which is ideal for a wheelchair user but which is situated on a steep hill miles from shops, the health centre and other facilities will allow independence at home, but is likely to hinder it in the wider environment.

The last decade has seen a tremendous upsurge in the building of sheltered housing schemes which offer the ideal for the elderly and disabled especially as help is available if necessary. These schemes fill a gap between totally independent living in their own homes and residential care.

Special housing schemes for disabled people have received a mixed reception from the general public, some having met with strenuous opposition from local residents, usually borne out of misconceptions about disability and illness, whereas others have been readily accepted. Nelson observes: 'the community or established group will resist most strenuously integrating newcomers who are different and who do not conform to accepted norms. It will, however, more willingly provide for those who are different but already part of their numbers.'[4] Thus the housing complex built for local elderly residents is likely to meet with community approval, because the elderly are a known part of our society and many people see themselves at that stage in the future. A sheltered housing scheme for mentally handi-capped people or a group home for rehabilitation of psychiatric patients is likely to meet with more opposition, usually because of ill-founded prejudices on the part of the community. Once such a scheme is established and functioning, local residents often wonder why they were initially opposed to it.

Housing can, but need not, be a barrier to independence if its design and necessary refurbishment are not carefully considered. The expertise of the occupational therapist liaising with both client and housing authorities is invaluable (see Chapter 9).

Education

The education of young people with a handicap is restricted more by architectural barriers than any other reason. Most schools are sadly lacking in facilities for disabled people, teachers as well as pupils. An additional problem is that children may require treatment sessions for medical and other problems whilst at school which reduces the time available for teaching. Only a few educational establishments are able to cope with these problems. The Warnock Report (1978) recommended that disabled children be integrated into normal schools. Unsuitable accommodation and lack of finance to alter the situation means that no significant progress has been made since the publication of the report.

Choice of further and higher education is also limited for many disabled people because of unsuitable buildings. Others find it difficult to attain the required educational standards for admission owing to schooling having been interrupted by intermittent hospi-talisation and/or illness. The Open University has been the channel of choice for many disabled people as it has opened up avenues previously closed to them. If educational opportunities are reduced so too are work opportunities especially in our current 'qualification conscious' society. Every effort must therefore be explored to improve the range of options available for disabled people in the field of education and minimise it as a problem in achieving independence.

Financial independence

Most people see work as a means of financial independence. In society today, work is at a premium which means that competition for available jobs is high. Disabled people generally have to prove themselves to be even more capable of work than non-disabled people, and in many cases they do not get that chance. Many people who are disabled have to rely on state benefits as they cannot work or are unable to cope with its demands whereas others are unable to find work.

The variety and complexity of the various benefits makes it very difficult for people to know to what they are entitled. Community staff must either know what benefits are available or know who to direct people to in order that they can be helped to apply for them. The Disability Alliance produces an excellent publication, *The Disability Rights Handbook*, which is reviewed annually. It contains help and advice about benefits including criteria for their award, how to apply and the amount of money involved.

Regarding finances, Blaxter comments, 'There are few people to whom a total disablement does not present some financial difficulty; to that extent, it is a function of the degree of impairment. To most people any long-term sickness or impairment means at the least some adjustment in their financial affairs. Yet one man's adjustment may be undreamed of wealth to another.'[5]

Many disabled and ill people have special needs which cost extra money, e.g. transport, dietary requirements and additional heating. It is important that they have sufficient money for these needs without having to limit spending on other essential requirements. Money does not buy health but it certainly helps to make illness and disability more tolerable. Lengthy discussions and complicated legislation can be very confusing to the disabled person and help may be needed to guide them through the labyrinth of bureaucracy. The therapist who will be more familiar with these procedures needs to show the utmost patience when discussing them. Written procedures to which reference can later be made will be of enormous help to the person and their family.

Society

To be totally independent, especially in fulfilling long-term goals for independence, requires co-operation and empathy from society as a whole. Society in general is unsure of how to react to disabled people; this is largely due to lack of opportunity, especially for meeting physically disabled people because of the vast environmental and architectural barriers that exist in our community. The reactions of non-disabled people on meeting those with a disability are variously described by Greenway and Harvey as 'over-solicitous, shifting attention away, focusing on anything irrelevant or becoming "moral" about disability.'[6]

In their fight for independence some disabled people are their own worst enemies because of their aggressive approach to genuine offers of help. This can effectively turn people against helping and colour their views of disabled people in general. Being independent is ideal, but a little help is invaluable at the right times, especially when accepted gracefully. It must be added that it takes a lot of faith in other people to ask for help from a complete stranger who is likely to feel obliged to try to help but who may have no idea how to. This problem consequently stops many disabled people going out without a companion, thus restricting their activities.

It is a vicious circle: disabled people are not able to get out and about because of architectural barriers and consequently the general public do not become acquainted and familiar with them. All these factors and others will influence the goals set and their achievement and must be considered when setting goals initially so that they are realistic and individual.

Assessment

Helping the disabled person to achieve maximum independence is dependent on accurate assessment of their total needs – physical, functional and social.

Physical assessment

The physical features of the clinical condition will often determine the degree of disability, handicap, rehabilitation necessary, and independence that can be anticipated. This will of necessity include function and capabilities. Sometimes significant improvement can be made by the provision of appropriate equipment, aids, splinting and other hardware, especially for the more severely disabled, whilst the teaching of different techniques is all that is necessary for those with minimal handicaps.

Functional assessment

This must include both the questioning and observation of tasks under consideration and include the disabled person and his carers. They all may state that they can manage – but how? Observation of the difficulties of one task may lead to the identification and realisation of difficulties with others.

Psychological assessment

Some consider that many disabled people's personal characteristics are the result of external factors and if the family is supportive and the social environment conducive, the outcome of rehabilitation is likely to achieve maximum independence. Lack of achievement may be associated with lack of personal drive and motivation as well as the possible absence of opportunities or support. There is no evidence that there are particular personality traits associated with specific physical disabilities, but certainly some conditions do have a direct organic effect upon the brain and the central nervous system, resulting in an association with changes in intellect and personality.

Those with painful joint conditions such as rheumatoid arthritis, restrict their activities to avoid pain. Physical disabiliy, whether painful or not, will undoubtedly induce a reactive depression in many. However, evidence does show that many of those with non-progressive severe handicaps (e.g. paraplegia) do eventually have a resilience leading towards a stable personality because they no longer have to struggle with acceptance of the handicap – they make the most of what they have.

Acceptance of the condition is of prime importance before any degree of independence can be achieved – and this acceptance must not only be by the person concerned, but by all those around him. There is also a correlation between educational levels and achievement, although this must be considered very guardedly by the therapist as deep frustration and other factors can hinder progress. A full psychological assessment can often give an indication regarding the possible outcome of rehabilitation and indicate the channel of management that is likely to give the best results.

Social assessment

The majority of possible problems are those related to the 'handling' of the disabled person – whether handicapped by a physical or psychiatric problem, and how much they are able to co-operate. Adequate social assessment can only be achieved if the whole family and others are involved. The assessment will be complex, with those concerned only telling the therapist what they want her to know and perhaps keeping the real key to the situation out of bounds. The involvement of professional colleagues may be needed to be brought in to help in this discovery. Following careful and sensitive assessment a positive approach towards rehabilitation can be made.

Reassessment

Assessment must not be seen as an isolated single episode – it must be a continuing sequence of reappraisals and reviews by all concerned, including the disabled person himself. It should be based on physical, functional, educational, psychological and social attainments.

Setting goals

Setting goals can only be done by professionals in collaboration with the disabled person himself and his family. By giving advice about what can be offered in the way of help and support, the occupational therapist can help the disabled person to determine what his or her goals should be after identifying needs and aspirations. Thereafter the whole group requires to work together to achieve independence for all concerned. Some professional people make the mistake of creating dependence by unconsciously making the disabled person rely on them and other support services rather than helping them to help themselves.

Whatever the disability, the occupational therapist has a key role in helping the disabled person to achieve maximum independence. This needs a careful, sensitive and holistic approach to the person's care. A cognitive attitude to solving problems presented by the disabled person is invaluable and helps to achieve realism throughout the entire rehabilitation process. The stages involved in the process are as follows:

1. Understand the complete problem, having taken into account all possible influencing factors. Assessment of the problem and the person's difficulties must be made in the light of functional abilities and lifestyle required.
2. Identify the goals to be achieved – both short and long term.
3. Determine the options available in achieving the goals.
4. Collect any necessary information and data for these options.
5. Explore the implications and consequences of each option.
6. Select a solution.
7. Plan for implementation.
8. Implement the plan/programme. The programme must be organised to achieve the maximum potential and may involve the following:
    (a) Teaching new techniques so as to achieve independence by maximising abilities and minimising handicaps.
    (b) Provision of necessary aids where techniques do not satisfactorily achieve the tasks required.
    (c) Advice on housing adaptations or selection to overcome environmental problems.
    (d) Development of intellectual stimulation and motivation in order to achieve a good quality of life.
    (e) Work with carers to enable normal interaction and relationships and maximise their independence.
9. The plan or programme must be evaluated and assessed to ensure that it is fulfilling the goals satisfactorily.

It is vital that this process is accomplished with the collaboration and co-operation of all professionals and other agencies involved with the disabled person. A team approach not only helps to resolve matters more quickly and with less effort than a series of individuals working towards similar goals in isolation, but is far less confusing to the individual and his family.

As already stated in Chapter 3, the community occupational therapist, especially if undertaking a generic role, needs to have a fund of knowledge to meet all the needs of those referred. This can be overwhelming and can encourage the notion of 'Jack of all trades and master of none'. This must not be the case. There are very special skills needed by community therapists which embrace shrewdness in identifying the person's *real* problem as early as possible and discerning whether and what kind of help is needed.

Time will be needed, first to gain the person's confidence, to build a rapport, and then to give him the time for learning new skills and life patterns as well as for counselling if this is needed. Working with people in their own homes requires more time than that required in other situations. It also requires time for the involvement of the family, as their lives could well be affected by possible changes to lifestyle.

The disabled person, and maybe his family, will need precise short-term and long-term goals – whether it be making a cup of tea, or getting back to work. Diffuse aims such as 'rehabilitation' and 'independence' are not helpful to any and often raise unrealistic expectations for the patient and family, although, more often than not, the patient will have unrealistic expectations. Unrealistic goals are also non-productive and demoralising for all concerned. However, helping the disabled person who is depressed, unmotivated and/or unrealistic to make and achieve their own goals is not only the most rewarding thing for the therapist, but the most important achievement in the rehabilitation process. The occupational therapist is trained in the art of motivation and helping the patient to gain insight; these skills therefore need to be used fully within a community setting. The concept of rehabilitation has been described as a form of 'behavioural therapy' and here again these skills and techniques need to be used and developed. The role of the occupational therapist in social skills training, behaviour modification, projective techniques and assertiveness training all play their part and can be achieved through specific treatment programmes as well as activities such as domesticity, creativity, work and recreation. The occupational therapist also needs to have the ability to restore or instil confidence within the disabled person, and the diligence to uncover talents that are obscure or hidden. The therapeutic programme should be time-limited, even if periodic reviews are needed. Ultimately, though, the aim for the disabled person should be to live in such a way that professional and medical advice is only sought as he/she wants it.

What must be fostered now and in the future is the idea of integration of handicapped and disabled people into a place in the community where they can lead the life they choose with as few barriers as possible. This can only be achieved by positive discrimination for disabled people which allows integration into all aspects of life, not just within their own homes, but also in schools, colleges, universities, work places, shops and public buildings. Through integration with able-bodied people disabled members will in turn lead to improved integration and the opportunities to achieve the level of independence to which each individual aspires.

References

1. T. Dartington, E. Miller, and G. Gwynne, *A Life Apart*, Tavistock Publications, 1981.
2. C. Safilios Rothschild, 'Disabled persons self-definitions and their implications for rehabilitation', *Handicap in a Social World*. A. Brechin, P. Liddiard and J. Swain, Eds, Hodder and Stoughton in association with the Open University, 1982.
3. M. Blaxter, *The Meaning of Disability*, Heinemann Educational Books, 1980.
4. R. Nelson, *Creating Community Acceptance for Handicapped People*, Illinois, USA, Charles C. Thomas, 1978.
5. M. Blaxter, op cit.
6. P. Greenway and D. Harvey, 'Reactions to physical handicap', in *Problem of Handicap*. (R. S. Laura, Ed.), The Macmillan Company of Australia Pty Ltd, 1980.

Chapter 6

Counselling

ELIZABETH CRACKNELL
Director of Training, School of Occupational Therapy, Northampton

An occupational therapist employed by a local authority social service department received a request from the local hospital to visit a 60-year-old man. Mr B had just been discharged home following an above-knee amputation and the request for a walking aid had come from a hospital department. The occupational therapist telephoned the hospital to find out a little more about the client and she was told that he had not progressed at all well in hospital – indeed there was nothing more that could be done for him as he was not making any effort. Mr B was being sent home to fend for himself as best he could. The occupational therapist was rather concerned at this so she arranged to go and see him at home that week. On arrival she found a very distressed person who looked far older than his years, together with a very anxious wife. Both were overwhelmed by the events which had overtaken them. His life had been turned up side down by the unexpected happenings – from an active, lively, confident man into an invalid (in-valid) who could not face his family, friends or the future.

The occupational therapist quickly realised that practical help in such circumstances was inappropriate and she spent the next one and a half hours listening to the outpourings of grief and anguish through tears as Mr B expressed all the pent-up emotions that consumed him and for which, since the operation, he had had no opportunity of release. In hospital the norm was to put on a brave face as practical difficulties were dealt with, for there was always 'someone worse off than you'.

This vignette of Mr B illustrates how essential it is for the community occupational therapist to be sensitive to all aspects of her client's being and not just respond to the presenting practical problems if she is really going to meet the needs of the individual. For this man, healing could only begin once the emotions surrounding his operation and permanent disability could be expressed fully. Someone had to give time, a listening ear, and understanding. Fortunately, the therapist recognised Mr B's state of distress, and psychological needs, and provided the opportunity that had not previously been available. After the first lengthy meeting he began to make good progress. Within a few weeks he looked ten years younger as he walked independently on his pylon, and began to plan for the future. An ostensibly practical referral for a man with a mobility problem was in reality a very different encounter, because the therapist responded to the client's psychological needs first and entered into a counselling relationship using very different skills.

The concept of counselling

Counselling is an activity which is carried out by many professional people as an integral part of their work as well as by those who are appointed to designated counselling positions. Clergy, teachers, managers as well as those in the helping professions often find that they are called upon to 'counsel' someone even though they may not feel adequately prepared for such a task. The demand for such help is growing and occupational therapists are increasingly aware of the necessity to learn *listening skills* in order to be effective in their work.

Most counselling occurs between two individuals, one person being in need of help and the other one the helper. The term counselling is often used loosely to refer to any help that is given by one person to another, such as advice, but strictly speaking such information giving is not counselling.

Counselling is a psychological process whereby one person helps another to explore feelings, thoughts and issues in life which are important to them. Through this exploration, recognition and discussion, the client is able to learn fresh ways of looking at events and of using his own resources to live more effectively. Counselling has been described as treatment;[1] however, this suggests a close link with the medical profession and patient passivity, but this is not so. It involves the person in his *own* development and change. Barry Hopson emphasises change in these words; 'Counselling is a process through which a person attains a higher stage of personal competence. It is always about change'.[2] Whereas another states that counselling aims to help clients who are mainly seen outside medical settings to help themselves.[3] None of these definitions are problem orientated, for many counsellors believe that the basic process has much deeper aims comprising greater independence, self responsibility and integration of the individual through growth and development. Carl Rogers, to whom the counselling world owes so much, emphasised that the individual should be the focus and not the problem. Thus the aim of counselling is not to solve one particular problem but to assist the person to grow, so that he or she can cope with present and future problems.[4] Rogers assumed that all have internal resources for understanding and changing themselves; that they can remain in control and be responsible for their own lives; and that they do not have to become dependent on others to be helped, for if they do, they lose their autonomy and impede the process of change.

From these definitions it can be seen that counselling and occupational therapy do have common features. Both activities emphasise the importance of the relationship established between the client and the therapist and both aim to help people to help themselves towards greater independence of living.

A holistic model

Counselling encompasses three major domains of a person's being:
1.   *Thinking*: the cognitive processes.
2.   *Feelings*: the effective processes.
3.   *Behaviour*: actions.
These three aspects of human functioning, together with the social relationships of the individual, constitute a holistic perspective of the person which is familiar to occupational therapists. This model is based upon the belief that psyche and soma are inextricably linked and both are affected by social events. Whatever happens in one domain will strongly influence the others. The depressed person will think, feel and behave in different ways from the way he behaved prior to the depression; similarly the person who is seriously injured will undergo changes in thoughts and feelings about himself, others and the world in general. This is shown diagrammatically in Fig. 4.

To treat one aspect and ignore the others will not cater for all the needs of the client and the neglected ones could interfere with the

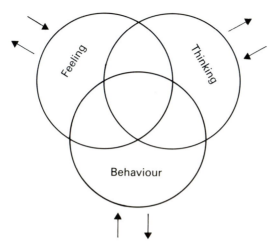

Fig. 4 Interactions.

process of healing. To treat the whole person the therapist must therefore include the psychological, social and physical needs of the individual if she is to be truly effective. This system is illustrated by Mr B. Such a dramatic occurrence as happened not only left him with a severe disability which seriously impaired his physical functioning, but it was a fact he had to come to terms with. Nothing would restore his leg to him; his body would be permanently incomplete and he knew that life for him would never be the same again. Inevitably things would change for he was no longer the man he once was. His *feelings* about himself and others had also changed. He no longer knew how others would receive him which made him anxious and uncertain. He did not like himself and believed that others would not like him in this condition either. His *thinking* became irrational as he felt he could no longer support his wife as he should and in fact felt useless and questioned the point of continuing life – for how could anyone possibly love him now? The occupational therapist found a defeated man. The amputation had changed everything about Mr B. His *behaviour*, of necessity, could no longer be as it was, as activity was limited, and his *feelings* and *thoughts* changed to attend only to the problem of physical limitations.

Humanistic theorists such as Maslow[5] and Rogers believe that each person has a unique perception of him or herself. The perception or self-concept comprises thoughts, feelings and values of the individual derived from past experience. Everything that happens to one is evaluated in relation to this self-concept. A person with a strong positive self-concept will view the world very differently from someone with a weak one. A man like Mr B may no longer feel good about himself, owing to his self-concept having changed. By listening to him and allowing him the chance to express powerful emotions, the therapist helped him to get in touch with some good things about himself and life which enabled reconsideration of who and where he was, and what options might be available to him. Only as that change began was it right for the occupational therapist to offer Mr B the practical help he required to assist his mobility, thereby extending his opportunities for action.

The counselling relationship and processes

No two people in a counselling encounter bring to it the same things. Each person has his or her own philosophy of life, personal values, attitudes and beliefs which affect the way all that happens is perceived. All events are interpreted in the light of previous experience and responses are based upon these perceptions. Where the people are very similar to each other, communication runs smoothly, but if they are very different, interaction may give rise to many misunderstandings as each views the world very differently. Both people convey and receive messages to and from each other in the specific context of place, time and relationship. The relationship is strongly influenced by the environment, and it will be noted that this will be very different in the home from that established by the occupational therapist in the hospital. Diagrammatically, the counselling process is seen as that shown in Fig. 5.

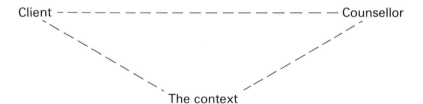

Fig. 5 The counselling relationship and processes.

The influence of the environment

Environmental psychologists who study the way places influence perceptions, attitudes and behaviour specify three important concepts which are relevant to community care.

The first concept is territoriality. The Englishman's home is his castle is a well rehearsed maxim. The house is where the major events of life occur, where residents sleep, eat, make love, celebrate, give birth and die. It is the place where the occupier has full control and where, under normal circumstances, entry is allowed only to those to whom permission has been given. It is the occupational therapist who is in a strange place, and not the client, and she is there only because permission has been granted to her.

The second concept is that of privacy – that is, the degree to which an individual allows access to himself, and how much he is willing to share and disclose. In hospital the patient has little say regarding matters of privacy. The power to exercise control there is in the hands of the hospital staff, who ask many intimate questions which every patient feels obliged to answer. In the home this situation is reversed. The client is independent of the services staff, he is directing his own life as much as possible, and is able to determine the extent to which he will allow the occupational therapist and others access not only to the house, but also to himself as a private citizen.

Personal space is the third concept. Edward Hall, an anthropologist, proposed the science of 'proxemics',[6] the way in which space is used in relationships and communication. Each person has a feeling of space around the body which they regard as their own and in which one feels comfortable. Cultural patterns vary, but for most of us if strangers come too near, particularly within eighteen inches, the intimate zone, it feels like an intrusion and can give rise to great discomfort. Treatment cannot be carried out from a distance. Members of the treatment team, who have no personal relationship with a patient from necessity, constantly violate this feeling of personal space which for some people causes distress and even anger. In the home the position is reversed. The client is the host and the roles demand patterns of behaviour whereby the therapist must be more circumspect and sensitive to the communications of the client if she is to gain his co-operation.

The characteristics of the relationship

Rogers proposed that there are three important ingredients which constitute a helping relationship irrespective of the theoretical orientation of the therapist. He defined them as *positive regard, empathy and congruence.* Truax and Carkhuff tested these three 'core facilitative conditions' extensively and found them to be essential for effective counselling.[7] Without these characteristics the process of counselling is not likely to prove very helpful and at times could be harmful.

Positive regard. The client in distress may behave very oddly, even in a bizarre fashion, have some funny ideas about himself and prove to be very unco-operative. Even so, it is important that he should be warmly accepted for who he is and valued as a person without conditions being applied or sanctions imposed. Acceptance does not mean approval. A person can be accepted without his behaviour necessarily being condoned. Such a quality is the mark of many friendships where one can like someone very much, but still dislike some of the things they do. The therapist who can accept the client in non-possessive, without judgement, and values him is more likely to provide the milieu for growth and change.

Empathy. Each person views the world from his or her own standpoint which is unique to him or her, and influences all the interactions with other people. The behaviour of others is likely to be interpreted in the light of this and assumptions are made based within one's own frame of reference. *To enter into a counselling relationship requires the counsellor to drop one's own view of the world and adopt that of the client.* To understand his story, the therapist counsellor has to be in tune with his experiences and feelings, enter his phenomenal field, and perceive events the way he does. Only then will the therapist be able to comprehend accurately and reflect what is happening to the client, and explore realistically what the possibilities are. Rogers states that empathy means entering the private perceptual world of the other and becoming thoroughly at home in it.[8] This will mean being sensitive throughout the sessions to the changing emotions of fear, rage, tenderness, confusion or whatever being experienced.

Congruence. In life, an individual may play many parts and at times one is conscious of putting on a front, or a façade which is not really oneself. Congruence means being genuine, sincere without a mask. Being true to oneself, and having the confidence to trust oneself freely, requires an authenticity of being which is the most problematical of these three qualities and depends to a large extent upon the therapist's own personal development. Congruence also means that the therapist has to be aware of her own personal responses within, and be comfortable with them, whatever they might be. She does not need to pretend to be anything other than she feels herself to be.

Listening and reflecting

Some people are thinkers, some are doers, and some are chatterers but to be a good counsellor one has to be a good listener. *Listening* is an art and skill which most people have at varying levels of competency, and one which can be developed with practice. It is defined as concentrating on hearing something and paying attention to it. It is a very active process, and involves not just attending to what is being said, but also observing how it is said. The body language conveys the feelings underlying the statements and due regard must be paid to both if one is really to listen. The aim must be to help the client to listen to himself, which requires sensitivity and patience from the therapist.

To listen accurately both should sit comfortably in a place where they are not likely to be disturbed. The therapist, focusing on the other person, must listen calmly as the client tells his story, which she interprets as far as she can from the client's standpoint and not from her own. She will need to attend to the expression of feelings, attitudes and beliefs as he recalls the events which have led him to be in his current position. Egan calls this the stage of exploration[9] – the period when the therapist is being put in the picture, listening to both verbal and non-verbal messages; checking, so that she knows she has understood the problem and asking for clarification when the story is confused.

A friendly manner, not an inquisitive one, will encourage the client to talk easily. As the therapist gathers the information she should then paraphrase what has been said and present her understanding of his experience to him. This reflection allows the client to listen again to the story he is giving, and correct any mistakes. It may encourage him to expand some points which do not convey the importance that they have for him, and it enables him to reflect upon his own words and position, which may help him to see ways forward, which at that time he was unaware.

Questions are useful but should be used with care. In basic listening exercises many students ask so many questions that the 'client' undergoes an interrogation, which leads to a clamming up rather than a flow of conversation. Open ended questions are likely to elicit more from the client than those which require a yes/no answer. 'Tell me what happened next' may lead to many unexpected things which the client is free to formulate as he wishes. A comment on the listener's observations, such as the restlessness when the client mentioned the doctor, may trigger some feelings in the client of which he was not wholly aware, and which he is now able to face.

The process of reflection mirrors for the client what he has said and enables him to experience more fully what is going on within him, and shows him that the therapist is responding, not from her own frame of reference, but has entered the client's phenomenal field. Together the two people move forward, often struggling hard to understand and be understood.

Establishing goals. Sometimes to listen attentively is all that is required of a therapist, but at other times it is necessary to discuss ways in which the client can move forward from his present predicament. What does he really want? And what actions is he prepared to take to change his position? In his distress he is unable to see a way forward but calmly and firmly the therapist may be able to make some suggestions. Here she may draw on her own experience, having much wider knowledge of available resources, but in no way must she impose her wishes upon the client. 'If I were you . . .' is a phrase which has no part in counselling. The consequences of any actions may be thoroughly discussed by both parties, but the decisions as to what goals should be set must stay with the client. At all times must he remain in control and be responsible for the decisions made and the actions that follow. However, he may need to rely heavily upon the therapist for support and guidance as he makes his moves.

Making decisions often leads to a reduction in tension, some relief, and releases energy and confidence, increasing the personal strengths upon which the client can draw. Through the experience the client develops greater integration as a person, develops more of his life independently in the future.

The therapist as an agent of change

A fundamental belief which underpins the practice of occupational therapy is that people can change, that one is 'never too old to learn'. Treatment is designed to increase all aspects of functioning as well as growth in confidence through the learning of new skills, in order that the client may lead a fuller life. A therapist must have a stong belief that individuals can change, for if she does not, she has little to offer her clients. She must also believe that people are important to themselves, and not for the positions they hold in society. Many clients are elderly and no longer command occupational status, but they are still important individuals, and need to be respected and valued as such. Therapists are like all other people in that they have problems and dilemmas, joys and sorrows in life, and like others, will have only partial awareness of their own motivations, attitudes and feelings. Those unknown processes can interfere in the relationship with a client, impeding the process of help. Bugental points out that the therapist's own emotions, conflicts, and anxieties will inevitably have an effect upon the client's life.[10] He was in fact writing about psychotherapy, but it equally applies to counsellors and occupational therapists. Thus the occupational therapist may find herself counselling a client hearing things that have never been put into words before, and she must respect these confidences. If for any reason she feels impelled to tell some other person, the client must be informed so that the trust placed in her is not broken. Wise judgement needs to be exercised, as the therapist weighs up the pros and cons of her decision. For someone who finds themselves undertaking much counselling work the support of a supervisor will be needed.

Community occupational therapists will visit many different people of varying ages, occupational groups, ethnic groups and backgrounds, and will meet a wide variety of problems. No two people are the same, for all have differing expectations, responsibilities and lifestyles. Consequently the needs of a person who is seeking help will be diverse and may be associated with any life event. In Holmes and Rahe's Social Adjustment Scale[11] the death of a spouse is the life event which causes most stress to the partner. Divorce is another change in life which creates stress, and when specific counselling help may be required. Physical disability may lead to problems with a person's sexual life, which can contribute to a crisis in the relationship.

Whatever the cause of distress and anguish, the basic principles of counselling are the same – i.e. the helper creates a warm, friendly, accepting atmosphere; listens attentively; reflects what she experiences to the client with emphatic understanding. In such a relationship the client is able to express emotions, develop new insights, explore possible avenues of action, make decisions and struggle forward.

References

1. P. Halmos, *The Faith of the Counsellors* London: Constable 2nd edn, 1978.
2. B. Hopson, 'Counselling and helping', in *Psychology for Occupational Therapists* (Ed. Fransella, F.), Macmillan, 1982.
3. R. Nelson-Jones, *Practical Counselling Skills*, Holt, Rinehart and Winston, 1983.
4. C. R. Rogers, *Counselling and Psychotherapy*, London: Constable, 1942.
5. A. H. Maslow, *Motivation and Personality*, Harper & Row, 2nd edn, 1970.
6. E. T. Hall, *The Hidden Dimension*, London: Bodley Head, 1966.
7. C. B. Truax and R. R. Carkhuff, *Towards Effective Counselling in Psychotherapy: Training and Practice*, Chicago: Aldine, 1967.
8. C. R. Rogers, 'Empathic: an unappreciated way of being', *The Counselling Psychologist* (Vol. 3, no. 2) pp. 2–10, 1975.
9. G. Egan, *The Skilled Helper*, Brooks Cole, 2nd edn, 1982.
10. J. F. T. Bugental, *Psychotherapy and Process: the Fundamentals of an Existential Humanistic Approach*, Reading, Mass: Adison-Wesley, 1978.
11. T. H. Holmes, and R. H. Rahe, 'The social readjustment rating scale', *Journal of Psychosomatic Research*, Vol. 14 pp. 391–400, 1970.

Further reading

L. M. Brammer, *The Helping Relationship Process and Skills*, Prentice Hall, 1979.

J. Brannen, and J. Collard, *Marriages in Trouble*, Tavistock Publications, 1982.

J. Dominian, *Make or Break, An Introduction to Marriage Counselling*, SPCK, 1984.

J. V. Dongen-Garard, *Invisible Barriers in Pastoral Care with Physically Disabled People*, SPCK, 1984.

M. Jacobs, *Still Small Voice, An Introduction to Pastoral Counselling*, SPCK, 1982.

E. Kennedy, *On Becoming a Counsellor*, Gill and Macmillan, 1977.

U. Kroll, *Sexual Counselling*, SPCK, 1980.

R. Nelson-Jones, *The Theory and Practice of Counselling Psychology*, Holt, Rhinehart and Winston, 1982.

C. R. Rogers, *On Becoming a Person*, London: Constable, 1967.

C. R. Rogers, *A Way of Being*, Boston: Houghton Mifflin, 1980.

P. Speck and I. Ainsworth-Smith, *Letting Go: Caring for the Dying and Bereaved*, SPCK, 1983.

W. Stewart, *Counselling in Rehabilitation*, Croom Helm, 1985.

Resources

The BBC tapes: *Principles in Counselling* obtainable from The British Association of Counselling, 37a Sheep Street, Rugby, Warwickshire CV21 3BX.

Helpful organisations

The Marriage Guidance Council, Herbert Gray College, Rugby, Warwickshire.

Cruse. An organisation which aims to relieve distress amongst the widowed. There are local branches in most areas.

Chapter 7

Which aid?

ANN MOY
Occupational Therapist, Norwich

An aid is a specially designed item of equipment intended to facilitate an activity – a tool for living. They range from something as simple as a knife with an enlarged handle to the complexities of electronic environmental control systems. Aids are frequently designed for a specific disability, often by the disabled person himself, or a specific activity, and it is often not until marketed are they found to have a wider application.

Too many aids however can become a hindrance rather than a help to the handicapped person, and therefore a careful assessment into their real needs must be made before any such equipment is issued or recommended. A research study[1] at Loughborough Institute for Consumer Ergonomics revealed that amongst 500 elderly and disabled people who had been provided with aids for assisting in every day activities the following usage was noted:

50% were not being used at the time of the study.
77% did not use their alarm system in an emergency.
29% bath aids were never used.
19% toilet aids were never used.
34% feeding aids were never used.

A further study undertaken by Lancashire Social Services[2] found that only 52% of all their aids issued were fully used, with over half the remainder never in use at all. Other studies have found similar trends and when investigated further the reasons not only revealed inappropriate recommendations but poor design and quality as well as inadequate training in their use and reassessments.

In many situations a new technique in achieving a required activity is far more appropriate than the provision of an aid in order to provide a quick solution to the presenting problem. An adjustment to an existing piece of equipment or furniture may also be a simpler and more acceptable solution – and indeed cheaper. For example, someone unable to exert sufficient pressure to cut up his food may find it easier if the table and chair were placed in a different position.

There is a growing interest in good design, so much so that at times it is difficult to identify between an aid and a standard piece of equipment – e.g. a jar opener which originated as an aid for the disabled person soon became a standard kitchen item obtainable in most hardware stores. Hence it is no longer considered an 'aid' in the original sense.

Improvement in design is growing as awareness of handicapped peoples' needs and realisation of the wider potential market is appreciated. Chairs, backrests, gardening equipment and telephones are just a few items which, because of good design, have become standard equipment suitable for many handicapped people. Consequently those with quite severe handicaps can now successfully use attractive standard equipment instead of the basic and utilitarian type previously designed specifically for them and thus identifying them as 'disabled'.

There will however always be those people for whom no alternative technique or standard piece of equipment is available and who require a specially designed aid. In these situations professional advice is essential as an incorrect choice can prove an expensive mistake and possibly detrimental to their condition.

The ultimate purpose of any aid, standard item or technique taught is to make an otherwise impossible activity possible, or a difficult one easier. If this objective is not achieved then the value of their introduction to the handicapped person will be lost. Where a person's condition improves or deteriorates regular reassessments will be necessary to ensure that the requirements are still being satisfied. Equipment no longer required should be removed as it may only take up valuable space and, in the case of deterioration of the condition, it may be a sad reminder of previous achievements.

Criteria for selection

Once it has been established that an aid is necessary four aspects should be considered before an actual choice is made:
1.   The disabled person's needs.
2.   The carer's needs.
3.   Objectives.
4.   Improvisation.

1. The disabled person's needs

An aid can only be of benefit when the handicapped person appreciates that it is needed. At first it may only be the physical aspect that he consciously recognises, but unless the psychological and social needs are also satisfied the aid may be quickly rejected. In fact some people are more willing to strive for physical achievement if an 'aid' is psychologically and socially acceptable to them! The occupational therapist must therefore carefully assess the handicapped person's needs before any issue of special equipment is contemplated.

2. The carer's needs

More often than not a carer is involved with the use of the more sophisticated aids such as a hoist. Their needs must be fully considered within the assessment.

3. Objectives to be achieved

The aid being considered must satisfy the objective for which it is being issued. For example, an electric page turner must allow for a book to be suitably positioned; however, if the prime objective was for the severely handicapped person who is an avid reader to read as many books as possible totally independently, then the choice should be one that he can operate himself and take a selection of different size books. Few suitable page turners are available and consequently it may be easy to recommend one at considerable cost to satisfy the demands of many people involved with caring for the reader, but owing to the limitations of the machine, the actual objectives could well not be met.

It is important to try the equipment in the intended situation, and for the activity in question, in order that all requirements are satisfied.

4. Improvisation using available equipment or materials

Many aids are considered by the general public to be expensive – a fact which is mainly due to a limited market for such specialised items. Adapted existing equipment therefore may well be considered as an alternative. Frequently it is possible for the occupational therapist assisted by a technician to improvise and adapt an existing aid and produce what is required at a fraction of the commercial price.

Choice of aid

The amount of choice that there is varies considerably depending on the activity to be achieved. For some, only one or two aids are available whilst for others a bewildering variety exists. A systematic approach for the consideration of any of the following aspects relevant to the aid in question should prevent unnecessary confusion.

1. Design or appearance

It is essential that the aid is aesthetically acceptable to the user and their family. Aids that are disliked are less likely to achieve their objective and be used regularly.

2. Method of control

Some aids are mechanically or electrically controlled. Where there is a choice of mechanism, such as in self-rise chairs or food whisks, the ability of the user must be carefully assessed to ensure that the item selected can be used safely and efficiently. The actual choice will depend on three equally important factors – the degree of disability of the user; their personal preference; and finance.

Mechanically operated aids usually require considerable hand and upper limb movement, the degree of necessary muscle power depending on the design. Electrically operated aids usually can be controlled by any part of the body – e.g. forehead, chin, elbow, knee (see Chapter 11). The amount of movement and muscle power required is minimal as long as the operating switch is positioned correctly.

3. Comfort

Pressure. The user and/or carer must be aware of any potential pressure points likely to be caused by the use of the aid. Such pressures can be caused by:

(a)   size of the aid;
(b)   shape of the aid;
(c)   type of material in actual contact with the user;
(d)   type of material beneath the surface – e.g. foam in cushions;
(e)   physical condition of the user such as bony prominences, sensitive skin, excess perspiration;
(f)   degree of muscle power required to operate the aid.

Position and posture. Maintenance of a correct posture is essential in order to achieve maximum performance as well as maximum well being. Considerations should include:

(a)   support of existing deformities;
(b)   elimination of spasticity;
(c)   quality of performance.

4. Safety

Stability. Specially designed furniture, standing frames and hoists should be sufficiently stable to enable the user to be left unattended for short periods of time. Back and front extensions to these, whilst assisting stability, can, if badly designed, create obstacles over which the user and others may trip (Photo. 1). An aid that is attached to a wall, floor, ceiling or item of furniture, must be firmly fixed and be able to withstand the amount of pressure or weight that is anticipated to be exerted on it whilst in use. The handicapped person and their carers must also have confidence in it.

Potential hazards. It is sometimes difficult to anticipate these as the most unlikely situation may suddenly occur thus causing a nasty accident. General aspects to look out for are:

(a)   sharp edges;
(b)   small apertures where fingers may get caught;

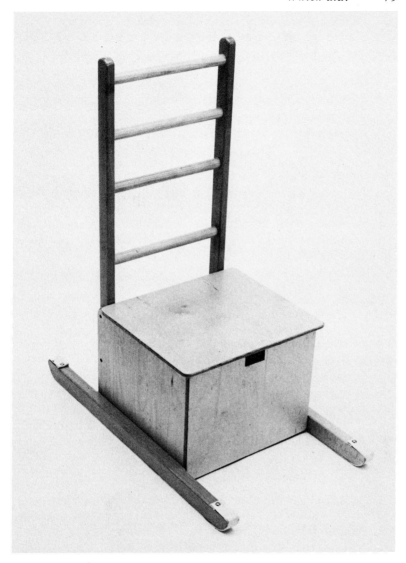

Photo. 1 An example of a child's chair with extensions to increase stability.

(c)   insecure collapsible or adjustable parts;
(d)   easily removable parts that may be dropped on the floor, mislaid or swallowed such as knobs;
(e)   exposed rods or poles;
(f)   required movements that are detrimental to the person's condition thereby contributing to pain and damage, e.g. rheumatoid arthritis;
(g)   inappropriate materials which may break whilst in use.

5. Durability

This should include consideration of both materials and methods of construction. Good design cannot hide inferior materials or workmanship and likewise unstable, shabby and badly designed equipment cannot be disguised by attractive materials and good workmanship.

6. Access

Ease of access to such furniture as tables, chairs, standing aids, prone boards and car seats is essential. It should be uncomplicated bearing in mind such times of emergencies as choking, fits, bleeding or fire. Difficulties in access may be caused by:
(a)   the height of the item;
(b)   the type of straps or other method of fastenings;
(c)   fixed or removable trays and tables;
(d)   methods of postural support or restraint other than straps, e.g. abduction blocks or angled seats (see Photo. 2).

7. Adjustments

Method. Various methods are used to adjust equipment such as pegs, screws and knobs. If alternative methods are available consideration should be given to:
(a)   how often the adjustments need to be made;
(b)   where the equipment is to be used and by whom;
(c)   how difficult the adjustment is to carry out and whether tools or assistance is required and if so whether they are accessible;
(d)   whether the user can remain in position whilst the adjustment is made.

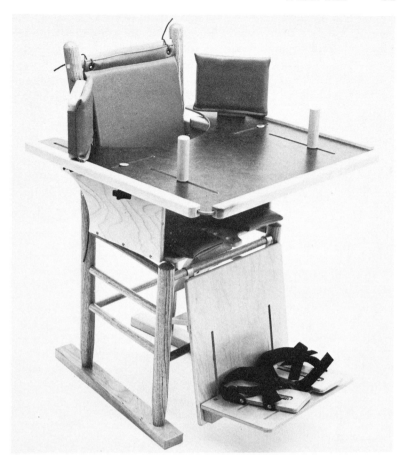

Photo. 2 Velcro straps and a quick-release mechanism on the tray allow a child to be quickly removed from this specially designed chair.

Range. Ensure that the range of adjustment is sufficient to accommodate the user's needs for a realistic period of time. For example, a person with a deteriorating condition may need to use an adjustable chair for at least 9–12 months.

Security. Ensure that:
(a)   the method of adjustment is secure throughout all positions;
(b)   the aid is stable throughout the full range of adjustment (often it can be unstable at either end of the range);

(c)   the means of retaining the adjustment. Some knobs and pegs can be accidentally removed or easily tampered with by another person, thus causing an accident. This is very relevant when children are around.

8.   *Weight*

This is especially important if the equipment needs to be transported regularly. A lifting handle, if one is available, will make this easier. However, if one is not present, a non-movable part that affords a secure grip should be identified. If the person responsible for carrying the equipment finds it difficult because of its weight or awkward shape a possible solution may be the provision of wheels or a trolley.

A large heavy aid that is usually stationary such as a special armchair may need to be moved occasionally for cleaning purposes. In most situations castors can assist in this but they should be those that have attached brakes.

A few aids such as electric hoists or stair lifts are permanently fixed and have moving parts. The weight is therefore not important to the user but to the structure supporting it, e.g. the ceiling or wall. It must be able to withstand the combined weight of the equipment and the user.

9.   *Dimensions*

The measurements or dimensions of the aid can be referred to as:

Standard. A non-adjustable aid designed to suit the average person. With some equipment such as the Rifton furniture for handicapped children more than one size is produced. Growth is therefore accommodated by a new item rather than by adjustment.

Adjustable. It is important to ensure that the degree of adjustment is adequate.

The dimensions of the selected aid, whether standard or adjustable, must not only meet the user's requirements but also allow him to be in a satisfactory position and a posture that is ergonomically correct for the chosen activity.

10. Transportation and storage

Many aids will be required in more than one place and thus will need to be carried around either regularly or occasionally. It may also be necessary to store them from time to time. The following points need to be considered if this is the case:

Foldability. Ease of folding or even dismantling an aid and how often this needs to be done.

Weight. This aspect has been considered in detail above.

Design. The shape, dimensions and type of materials used are all design features which need to be considered in relation to transporting and storing them. Particular features are:
(a)   extensions or any irregular shapes;
(b)   overall height, length and width of the item when folded;
(c)   type of material used;
(d)   movable and removable parts, e.g. footrests, table sur-rounds, slings. Care must be taken that no parts are lost;
(e)   carrying handles can be an advantage if well designed and in a convenient position.

11. Cleaning

Inaccessible cracks and corners that collect dust and dirt are a menace. Smooth, rounded or continuous surfaces help to facilitate cleaning.

The type of surface also facilitates ease of cleaning. Equipment used by several children or mentally handicapped people will need more frequent and harder cleaning than those used by one fastidious adult. Thus a work surface that will stand up to regular and hard cleaning should be chosen.

Fabric and padding should be removable and easy to clean and dry.

12. Maintenance and repairs

All aids and equipment should be well maintained in order to keep performance at its peak. The frequency of maintenance and repairs due to normal wear and tear can be anticipated, but equally accident, misuse and abuse must not be forgotten. Many firms will provide their own maintenance service and these details need to be known before the issue to a handicapped person. Agreement as to who should be responsible for the payment of these contracts also needs to be identified before issue. Many social service departments will agree to undertake this.

If the need for maintenance and repairs frequently occurs it may be due to an incorrect assessment.

13. Availability

Delay between selection and receiving the aid can prove a source of much anxiety and frustration to the person eagerly awaiting its arrival. Delivery times vary and are not always reliable. If the aid is urgently required the setting up of an aids library can prove a valuable solution (see Chapter 11).

Certain items are only manufactured on demand, or the person may need a specially designed piece of equipment designed to his individual specifications. In these cases 2–3 months should be allowed for delivery. Local REMAP groups may also come to the rescue.

14. Price

Prices vary from one manufacturer to another for what may appear to be identical items. Some catalogues state prices excluding VAT, postage and packing, whereas others include these additional costs. VAT can in some instances be avoided if a letter from the handicapped person's GP, stating that the equipment is essential, accompanies the order. However, the occupational therapist must be aware of changing legislation in this context.

Factors influencing acceptance

All the above factors will influence the handicapped person, his or her family and carers in whether or not the specially prescribed piece of equipment is acceptable. However, further major factors cannot be forgotten:

1. Suitability for use

This is sometimes difficult to assess unless the aid is available for a trial period in the intended situation and with all concerned. The aspects to consider are whether or not the aid is:

Functional. As well as being aesthetically acceptable it must achieve one or more of the following:
(a) enable the user to carry out a previously impossible activity;
(b) enable the user to carry out a previously difficult activity more easily;
(c) allow more enjoyment or sense of achievement;
(d) increase independence or lessen dependence;
(e) improve quality of life;
(f) improve the lot of the carer.

Efficient. The aid should enable the activity to be carried out with ease within the required period of time and to an agreed or acceptable standard.

Reliable. The aid should be capable of regular use and consistently achieve the required results. Frustration in its inefficiency resulting in lack of confidence in it, or perhaps eventual physical harm, can result in the aid not being used. More important, the handicapped person requiring this help will get more and more despondent.

2. Training in the use of the aid

However basic and straightforward the aid may be, it is important that either verbal or written instructions are available relating to the correct assembly, use and care.

A training session must always be included so that the user, carer and anyone else involved are fully aware of the aid's purpose and potential. These sessions should be carried out in the intended place of use or realistically related to it. Aspects to cover are as follows.

Preparation. For example:
(a) correct assembly (slings correctly positioned on the hoist)

(b)   correct adjustment (height and angle)
(c)   secure adjustment (knobs and screws tightened)
(d)   secure attachment (to table or bed).

Use. For example:
(a)   routine for access (transferring to bath seat from wheelchair and vice versa)
(b)   routine for required activity (establish movements within the capabilities of the user or carer which will achieve the required objective).

Care. As commented above.

3.   *Convenience for others within the same environment*

Other persons involved may be members of the family, pupils and staff at school, or staff in a day centre. Whatever the situation all involved should fully understand the need for the aid being provided. Also they should not be inconvenienced by it. Therefore to ensure that it is acceptable it should not be:

Disliked by other people, e.g. a fixed toilet seat may not be welcomed by other members of the family having to use the same toilet.

A disturbance to other people, e.g. the continual use of a noisy toy, or squeaky moving parts.

A hazard to other people, e.g. a young child can easily cause damage to himself, another person or an object if allowed to 'play' in an electric wheelchair belonging to another member of the family.

The occupational therapist should always try to consider who could be inconvenienced or harmed by any aid being recommended and how such an incident could be avoided before it occurs.

Factors influencing the rejection of an aid

1.   *Personality*

Like any other everyday piece of household equipment, an aid may be rejected due to the user's personal likes and dislikes. A flamboyant colour or modern design might be totally unacceptable to one person whereas acceptable to another. The occupational therapist must not be persuasive but should acknowledge these preferences.

2. Family influence

It is unlikely that the aid will continue in use if it is disliked by the family and friends especially if not fully understood or appreciated by them.

3. Lack of perception

If the reason for providing an aid is not recognised by all concerned and the benefits realised, then minimal effort will be exerted into its use. For example, mobile arm supports may not be readily accepted if the user is unable to reach all corners of his artist's pad.

4. Mental handicap

A mentally handicapped user may not have sufficient concentration, will power or mental ability to persevere with an aid particularly if the initial training is inadequate. In some situations an award system or achievement chart might encourage them and help to achieve the required results.

5. Time lapse

If the period of time between the onset of the disability and the commencement of the rehabilitation programme is too long then the person involved may:
(a)   become too dependent on the family or carer;
(b)   develop a method for coping with a situation which may encourage movements contradictory to progress;
(c)   become disinterested or disillusioned, making it difficult for the therapist to encourage their full participation in a treatment programme involving any necessary aids.

6. Inadequate assessment

Perhaps the most important factor. All necessary information relating to the intended activity to be achieved must be gleaned before any aid is considered. Although a standard procedure can be compiled for the assessment each situation must be considered individually.

7.   Lack of training

As indicated above.

8.   Lack of follow up and/or reassessment

Few situations remain constant for any length of time and therefore it will be necessary to arrange a follow up appointment to confirm that the equipment still satisfies the requirements of the handicapped person.

An 'aid' has been defined as being 'something that helps' and if any item does not fulfill this objective then it is, in fact, not an 'aid' to the person requiring it but a thorough nuisance.

References

1. M. Page *et al. The use of technology in the care of the elderly and disabled: Tools for Living*, London: Pinter, 1980.
2. S. Barrow and M. E. Derbyshire. *Survey on the usefulness of aids*, Lancashire County Social Service Department, 1975.

Further Reading

Ann Darnbrough and Derek Kinrade, *Directory of Aids for Disabled and Elderly People*, Cambridge: Woodhead–Faulkner, 1986.
DHSS 'Aids Assessment Programme'. Reports available from DHSS Store, Health Publications Unit, No. 2 Site, Manchester Road, Heywood, Lancashire OL10 2PZ
   Assessment of long handled reachers.
   Assessment of self-rise chairs and cushions.
   A comparative assessment of three types of moulded body supports.
   Office seating for the arthritic and low back pain patients.
   Assessments of back rests for use in car seats.
   Assessment of replacement car seats.
   Wheelchair cushions.
   Assessment of furniture designed for handicapped children.
   Assessment of feeding aids for handicapped children.

Incontinence aids for handicapped children.
Assessment of toilet aids for handicapped children.
Food preparation aids for those with neurological conditions.
Food preparation aids for rheumatoid arthritis patients.
A community study of the performance of incontinence garments.
Equipment for the Disabled Publications, Nuffield Orthopaedic Centre, Windmill Road, Headington, Oxford.

Resources

Disabled Living Foundation, 380/384 Harrow Road, London S9 2HU.
Local aids centres.

Chapter 8

Mobility

JANE R. PAGE
Community Physiotherapist, Aylsham, Norfolk

SUSAN BADDELEY
Occupational Therapist, Norwich

The importance of mobility for the physical and psychological well-being of disabled people is well recognised. It enables them to achieve greater independence and, in consequence, become integrated into society. Being mobile allows the person to make decisions and choices for himself and the opportunity to choose what he wants to do and when to do it.

Walking is a learned skill dependent on the ability of the central nervous system to control posture, balance and co-ordinated movements. Difficulties arise from many possible causes such as the hemiplegic person who may have interference with postural reflexes, loss of movement or change in muscle tone. Balance may be disturbed by lesions of the cerebellar, visual or vestibular systems. Loss of mobility may be the result of weakness in the trunk or lower limbs and this together with any change in tone will seriously affect posture and gait.

Walking ability is also associated with mental alertness but many physical factors such as joint degeneration and sensory deficit can also seriously affect it. Therefore when assessing the person who has mobility problems all these factors need to be noted and borne in mind when considering transfers and all daily living skills.

Obviously there are varying levels of mobility and some people may rely heavily on their carer to help them get about. In such cases the well-being of the carer is most important and must therefore be included in any assessments.

Mobility can help to prevent many physical difficulties such as bladder and bowel problems. It also assists in maintaining strength, range of movement and normalisation of muscle tone.

Enabling a disabled person to become mobile calls for a team approach. The physiotherapist will assist with gait patterns and exercise, the chiropodist with any appropriate care required, whilst the occupational therapist will assess for any necessary aids and adaptations. Between them they must aim to achieve the maximum potential function of the disabled person, giving consideration to his needs as well as those of the carer.

Although much has been written on mobility (see Further Reading), the following outlines some of the key factors that need to be considered by all community therapists in the assessment and maintenance of mobility, ensuring that safety within the home and surrounding environment is paramount.

Mobility in the home

More often than not the patient's home environment is far from ideal for increasing and maintaining mobility. The general design, with awkward corners, steps and thresholds often impedes progress, and the positioning of furniture, mats and electrical flexes create other hazards. Although some of these problems can be overcome by tactfully persuading changes in the home, some decisions will have to be made, resulting in a compromise. When assessing for mobility, consideration must also be given to the needs of those living within the same home, including children, and again some compromises may need to be made.

Hazards in the home

1.   Different floor coverings throughout the home can make the passage from room to room difficult. This may be solved by ensuring that the edges of carpets are well tacked or stuck down and that the lighting is improved.
2.   Loose carpets and rugs. If possible these should be removed or attached firmly to the underlying carpet.
3.   Poor lighting, especially in hallways, passages and stairs.
4.   Electrical flexes. Wherever possible extra plugs should be installed otherwise the flex should be tacked down.

5.   Animal feeding bowls, litter trays and baskets. These should as far as possible be kept to one side out of the normal walking path.

6.   Furniture with splayed legs. These need to be positioned in such a way so as to cause the least hazard.

7.   Low furniture and objects which may not be seen by the poorly sighted, e.g. footstools, radio placed on floor.

Education of the family and other carers may be necessary here.

Many patients, particularly the elderly, may rely on using furniture to get about and stability of these needs to be checked. Where there is an open fire the use of a fireguard is essential if the patient is unsteady on his feet.

The location of the toilet will be very variable. Many homes still have an outside toilet which may well not be situated adjacent to the house. This then will bring into question outside access and the condition of paths. A commode may be found to be a temporary solution, especially during bad weather, until alternative arrangements can be made. The question of emptying these however can pose problems. Chemical toilets may be supplied as these need emptying less frequently.

Steps and stairs

It may be possible to remove small internal thresholds or fit a small ramp at these. Care must be taken that any ramp however shallow will not interfere with the passage around the house and that it is fixed very firmly. Unfortunately, owing to limited access, steps between rooms can rarely be ramped. A half step or suitably placed handgrip may assist the handicapped person in these situations. This also may apply to outdoor steps. In both cases any half step, which is fixed or movable, must be large enough to accommodate the user safely with their walking aid.

When stairs can be negotiated but a walking aid is required methods of transporting the aid will need to be considered. In some cases two items may have to be supplied, one being left within easy access on either floor of the house.

Stairs can be a problem to some people. If they are unable to negotiate these even with the help of banisters either side, it may be feasible to instal a stair lift or even a home lift. These are extremely expensive and careful thought therefore needs to be given as to their suitability. Discussion needs to take place with local authority personnel as to funding possibilities for these, remembering that regular maintenance will be required.

Care of feet and footwear

The chiropodist should be involved with the care of feet particularly when there is discomforture. Observation and advice regarding correct footwear is essential especially for those with walking difficulties. Slippers and soft shoes should be strongly discouraged as they tend not to fit correctly and in consequence create a shuffling gait resulting in accidents. There is also the tendency for the foot to go sideways over the heel. Both these things cause uneven wear of the shoe which in itself can be dangerous.

Ideally shoes should be comfortable, well fitting, fairly highly cut and with a low heel.

Walking aids

It may be necessary for a person to use a walking aid in order to achieve or maintain independent mobility. The walking aids most commonly used are as follows:

1. walking sticks;
2. quadruped;
3. walking frame;
4. elbow crutches;
5. axillary crutches.

The purpose of the aid is to increase stability for those whose balance is affected, or have lost confidence in walking. This may be due to generalised weakness; a specific condition such as hemiplegia, multiple sclerosis, osteoarthritis; or as a consequence of surgery. For those who need to be partially or totally weight-bearing, as in the case of fractures of the lower limb, some or all of the weight will be taken by the arms through the walking aid. The use of the appropriate aid increases the size of the weight-bearing base thus producing greater stability (Fig. 6).

It is important that the person be correctly assessed, an appropriate aid provided, and adequate instruction given on its correct use and maintenance in order that maximum mobility and safety is achieved. In areas where there is a community physiotherapist it is usually their responsibility to do this.

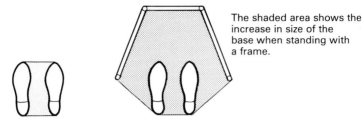

The shaded area shows the increase in size of the base when standing with a frame.

Fig. 6 Diagram showing the increase in size of the weight-bearing base when freestanding (left) and with frame (right).

Measurement for a walking aid

For a walking aid to be used properly it should be of the correct height. Careful measurements must be taken (see Photos 3a and 3b).

When the person is standing in an upright position he should be able to hold the required aid with his elbow in a comfortable position of 10–15° flexion. This can be achieved if he stands upright with his arm hanging loosely by his side. The measurement is then taken from the styloid process of the ulnar to the ground at a point 6 inches lateral to the heel of the shoe.

For maximum safety disabled people should be taught the care of their walking aid. Rubber ferrules must be checked regularly and replaced when showing signs of wear. Screws and nuts on walking frames must be kept tight and rust free. The occupational therapist can assist by teaching the family and others to routinely check these aids for wear and tear.

Walking aids in common use

1. *Walking stick*. Metal sticks have the advantage over wooden ones in that they are adjustable, whereas the latter are considerably cheaper.

Advantages. It is cosmetically acceptable; takes up little space during use and in storage; can easily be used on steps and stairs; is an aid that cannot be leant upon too heavily; one hand could be free to carry any necessary items and yet they can be used in pairs.

Disadvantages. It may not give enough support.

Shooting sticks, especially those in which the handle forms a foldaway seat, can be invaluable to those who need occasional or regular rests whilst out walking.

2. *Quadruped.* These may be advised when slightly more support is needed.

Advantages. They are particularly useful for amputees as an intermediate stage during the transition between a frame and two sticks. Here they should be used in pairs. They also provide greater stability than a stick whilst enabling a more normal walking pattern.

Disadvantages. It does not actually give much more support than a stick; it is clumsy and heavy; the user may trip over its 'feet' when in use; the user may become dependent on it.

3. *Walking frames.* These are generally used by elderly people. They can be fixed in height or be adjustable.

Advantages. The most stable form of walking aid provided it is used correctly with all four feet firmly placed on the ground together; it can be very light in weight; it provides symmetrical support.

Disadvantages. No hands are left free to carry any necessary items; it may be too wide to go through narrow doorways and between furniture; it is impossible to use on stairs and therefore it may be necessary for the disabled person to be provided with two frames, one to keep both upstairs and downstairs; where a person has already developed a poor gait pattern the use of a frame will not help in re-educating the gait pattern, however, confidence may be gained; there may be a tendency to take several steps carrying the frame – if so, the prescription is incorrect.

4. *Elbow crutches.* These are seldom supplied to those living in the community except following surgery or trauma when they may be given on discharge from hospital for the period of partial weight bearing.

5. *Axillary crutches.* Again these would seldom be supplied in the community except to those post-surgical or trauma patients who need to be non-weight bearing.

The occupational therapist must know what method has been taught and reinforce this by regular encouragement.

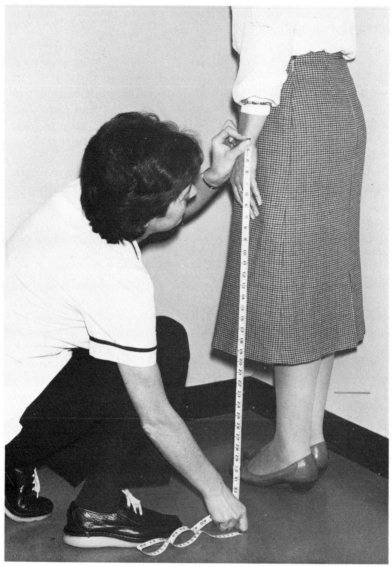

Photo. 3a Measurement for a walking aid.

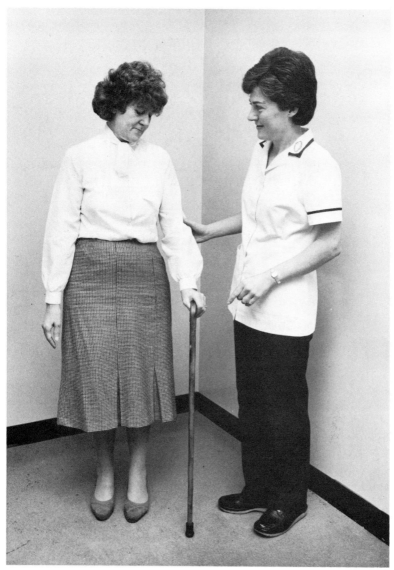

Photo. 3b Testing a walking aid.

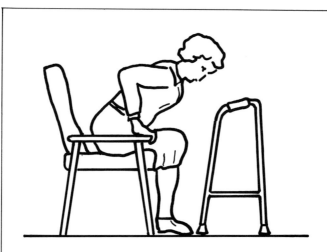

Getting out of a chair

1. Put your hands on the arms of the chair.

2. Place your feet flat on the ground, under your knees.

3. Lean forward so that your head is over your knees.

4. Move towards the front of the chair.

5. Keep leaning forward, and push with your hands on the arms of the chair to help you stand up.

Fig. 7 A sample instruction leaflet.

Methods of transfer

Teaching the patient to transfer themselves from one position to another follows similar principles.

1. *Sitting to standing.* Ensure that the walking aid is to hand; ensure that the body weight is well forward over the feet in order to minimise the effort required; place hands on the arms of chair, edge of bed or appropriate hand grip in toilet; lean forward to bring head in line with knees; keep leaning forward and push up with hands to the standing position.

An instruction leaflet (as that shown in Fig. 7) has been found to be of use in reminding the disabled person of the above sequence after the therapist has left.

2. *Standing to sitting.* Walk right up to the chair, toilet or bed and turn round; feel for the surface of the seat against the back of the legs; then, placing the hands on the chair arms, grab rails or bed edge, lower oneself gently to the sitting position.

It is important that if a person has difficulties with transfers all necessary items of furniture such as chair-bed and toilet are at compatible optimum height.

Chair

It is important that the disabled person not only has a comfortable chair in which to sit, but one which also maintains good posture and gives adequate support. If the chair in regular use is unsuitable there needs to be some careful persuasion to change to a more suitable model. If no such chair is available the existing one may then need to be adapted. This may include the use of chair blocks but again safety must be carefully considered. Fixed leg extensions, or a platform on which the chair can be fixed, may be the safest solution, although great care must be given to its design.

A solid base under the cushion encourages an improved sitting position and will make rising from the chair easier. This can be achieved by a board, firmer cushion, or, as a very temporary measure, a thick layer of newspapers.

Bed

The position of the bed is of paramount importance in facilitating mobility. It should be positioned in such a way as to allow easy access for the disabled person and his carer. If a wheelchair is to be used then the layout of the whole bedroom needs careful planning.

When considering transfers on and off the bed it is important to ensure its stability, the degree of firmness of the mattress and the correct height. The optimum height for a bed is 18 inches.

A firm base to the mattress enables ease of movement and assists rising to a standing position. A wooden board inserted between the base of the bed and the mattress will help to achieve this.

Toilet

The toilet, especially if in a separate room, is often a difficult place in which to manoeuvre particularly with walking aids or wheelchairs.

The door more often than not causes an obstruction. Possible solutions to overcome this are the rehanging of the door to open outwards, or fixing a sliding one.

As with beds and chairs, the height of the toilet needs to be compatible.

Toilet frames and grab rails strategically placed either side of the toilet may assist certain handicapped people to stand and balance whilst adjusting their clothing. Frames should be checked for stability and only used when the user is able to push with his weight placed evenly on both sides. Rails need to be carefully sited so that the user can *push* himself up from the seat to a standing position rather than pulling on the rail.

When access to the toilet is impossible or inadvisable a commode may be a solution. Again, stability of these must be checked and assessment regarding the type of commode will be required to determine whether or not arm rests and/or a backrest is required.

Wheelchairs

For some people a wheelchair is an essential mobility aid and therefore should not be seen as a badge of disability. It may be the only means for the disabled person to become more independent and participate in many additional activities by conserving energy that would otherwise have been exhausted by walking. Wheelchair mobility can make the difference between being confined to one room or being able to move throughout the home to employment, the school classroom or leisure pursuits.

The supplying of a wheelchair, however, is not necessarily the answer to all mobility problems and it is important that the disabled person and relatives realise the limitations that a wheelchair may have. A chair may in fact be contra-indicated if it is felt that it will discourage a patient from walking when this would be a necessary activity to help prevent further medical problems such as contractures and kidney problems. In these cases a wheelchair, if required at all, should only be issued for outdoor use.

Wheelchairs are categorised as follows:
1. Self propelling folding chairs.
2. Rigid chairs (suitable only for indoor use).
3. Folding push chairs.
4. Electrically propelled.

The first three categories can be prescribed by registered medical practitioners. For electric chairs, however, an assessment by the medical officer at the local artificial limb and appliance centre (ALAC) will be required. Assessment by the occupational therapist for the correct wheelchair must include the home situation and other relevant factors. Follow up on delivery will ensure that it is not only the correct model but will enable any necessary adjustments to be made, e.g. footplates, and to teach the user and the carer how to use the chair correctly. This session should include the importance of applying the brakes and raising the footplates before the patient sits or stands from the chair, and ensuring that the tyres are kept at the correct pressure. If the chair is to be used outdoors, the easiest methods of negotiating kerbs and slopes need to be taught. Finally the carer will need to be shown how to open and close the chair, and if necessary, the best method of getting it into their car.

The types of chair issued by the DHSS are clearly listed in the *Ministry Manual* (MUM 408) which is obtainable from: The Manager, DHSS Store, No. 2 Site, Manchester Road, Heywood, Lancashire OL10 2PZ.

This manual also includes a list of accessories that are available. Chairs can be adapted to accommodate specific problems and this is usually done in conjunction with the local technical officer or at the local wheelchair clinic.

Finding the most suitable wheelchair may be difficult as what is ideal for the disabled person may present problems to the carer and not be suitable within the environment. A compromise may therefore be necessary in order to find a chair that will suit all needs.

Assessment

Assessment is essential in order to supply the correct wheelchair. The following are the main points that must be considered:
The user
(a)   weight/height;
(b)   posture;
(c)   diagnosis – permanent/temporary use.
Who is going to propel the chair and how?
(a)   user;
(b)   carer;
(c)   user and carer.

Ability to self propel the chair
(a)   size and position of wheels;
(b)   type of tyres;
(c)   weight of chair;
(d)   ability to grip handrims.
Ability to push the chair
(a)   carer's age and health.
Home and outside environment
(a)   doorwidths;
(b)   turning spaces;
(c)   heights for transfers;
(d)   access;
(e)   local terrain.
Use of the chair
(a)   domestic;
(b)   leisure;
(c)   school;
(d)   work;
(e)   transportation.
Comfort
(a)   cushions;
(b)   seat size;
(c)   time delay.

Accessories

Accessories can add to the comfort and safety of the patient.

Cushions. These should always be ordered and thought given as to whether a baseboard would encourage a better sitting position. Special cushions are available to help prevent pressure sores and can be ordered through the DHSS but the more expensive of these, e.g. Roho Cushion, may require assessment at a clinic.

Trays. It is worth remembering that these usually need assembling after delivery, a task which may prove too difficult for the handicapped and elderly person to achieve himself.

The personal handbook issued with each wheelchair gives details of home maintenance and whom to contact if serious problems occur. A bicycle pump needs to be supplied for the chair tyres, and the valve at the end of the pump may need changing in some cases. Instruction about this is sent with the chair.

Electric powered wheelchairs

Electric powered wheelchairs supplied by the DHSS and operated by the handicapped person are only for indoor use, or for use in the immediate surroundings of their home. Attendant operated electrically powered chairs are available to help the carer if they are unable to manage a manual model. These have considerable limitations especially when negotiating steps and kerbs, and they are unable to negotiate hills. All of these chairs necessitate having somewhere dry to house them with an electric socket nearby for charging the battery.

Anyone considering purchasing any type of chair privately should be encouraged to seek expert advice and try several different models before making a final decision.

Ramps

The ideal gradient for a ramp is 1 : 20 but in practice it is often not possible to have such a long shallow ramp. The maximum gradient for a wheelchair to be self propelled or pushed is 1 : 12. Ramps should have a non-slip surface and a lip at the edges for safety.

Mobility in the environment

However well one is able to get around one's own home, mobility within the community can pose considerable difficulties. The home, to a certain extent, can be modified and adapted, but it is virtually impossible to alter the surrounding environment. Differing problems will be found depending on how much district councils are aware of the needs of handicapped people. The community occupational therapist should endeavour to facilitate changes.

Check list of possible problems

1. Gravel or uneven pathways and drives. It may be possible to have these tarmacademed and surfaced with concrete slabs.
2. Kerbs. Particularly when using a wheelchair, the use of driveways to cross roads is worth the extra steps required.

3.   Uneven pavements. Care needs to be taught in order to prevent tripping.
4.   Slopes/hills. These may be difficult for the wheelchair user. For short steep slopes it may be preferable to descend backwards.
5.   Obstructions, e.g. work being carried out to a pavement. This may be a particular problem to the visually impaired.
6.   Location of shops. Those may be too far away for the disabled person to get there and back with ease. Routes should be taken where there are seats or convenient walls to perch on en route.

Driving

The ability to drive despite a disability can mean that the handicapped person has considerably more control over his environment and lifestyle. The medical practitioner has the responsibility of saying whether or not they are fit to drive and he may ask the community therapist to give her opinion, particularly of cognitive function.

It may be that a car with automatic transmission and, possibly, power-assisted steering may be all that is required. However, much can be done to adapt cars to compensate for physical limitations and all should be advised to seek expert help. The mobile mobility centre recently set up by Banstead Place tours the country and offers assessment and advice to would-be car drivers.

Transfers/access. The width and height of the car door will be a factor determining the case in which the disabled driver or passenger can get in and out of a car. The angle of the open door may also be a crucial factor if transfers are made from a wheelchair, particularly if help is required. A simple sliding board may be all that is needed for this; however, special car seats and hoists may need to be considered.

Car hoists. A portable hoist, such as those used in the home, may be used to get the disabled person in and out of a car. Hoists which fit to the roof of the car like a roof rack are also available. These are extremely efficient and relatively easy to use. However, they would usually be regarded as an aid that patients would have to fund for themselves.

Car seats. Specially designed seats can be fitted in place of the original one on either the driver or the passenger side. They rotate through 90° and some models also slide forward in order to allow easier transfer (see addresses at end).

Adaptations. Many car conversions are possible and include:
(a)   hand controls;
(b)   steering knobs;
(c)   joystick steering;
(d)   gear lever knob;
(e)   key grips;
(f)   switch extensions.
For more details of these and addresses of suppliers, the Banstead Place Mobility Centre should be contacted.

Specially designed cars

Some cars are able to be converted in order to take a handicapped passenger in his wheelchair. This may mean raising the roof and installing extra side windows. A tail-lift will need to be fitted or at least a ramp into the car. Few people actually propel themselves up the incline unless it is a very low loader and therefore a strong pusher will be needed.

Garages

The siting and size of the garage or carport is important. More room is needed for a disabled person to get in/out of the car particularly if using a wheelchair. Car ports may be found to be more convenient.

Mobility allowance

This is a non-means tested, tax-free allowance, paid to those who are unable or virtually unable to walk. It is available from the age of 5 years and clients must have claimed this allowance before their 66th birthday. Limitations may be imposed on the length of time that clients can receive this; however, in some cases, it can be paid until the 75th birthday.

To qualify for the mobility allowance clients must be unable, or virtually unable, to walk and are likely to be in that condition for at least one year. The occupational therapist should become familiar with the current regulations. People with mobility difficulties due to psychiatric illness or mental handicap may also be able to claim this allowance.

If an application is turned down it is always worth considering appealing. In this case it is helpful if the therapist can send a detailed report as to the client's ability and problems. A useful checklist which can form the basis of a report is published by the Disablement Income Group Charitable Trust (DIGCT). This trust has an advisory service which offers information and advice on the full range of financial provisions available to disabled people.

Motability

Motability was established in 1978 as a voluntary organisation. It was set up, supported by the Government, in order to help people who were in receipt of the mobility allowance to lease or buy on hire purchase a car or an outdoor electrically powered wheelchair. Some financial help may also be available to help adaptations to the cars. Details of the scheme are available from: Motability, Boundary House, 91–93 Charterhouse Street, London EC1M 6BT (Tel. 01-253 1211).

Orange badge scheme for disabled and blind people

This national scheme allows holders of the badge to be exempt from certain traffic regulations for the purpose of car parking. Issue is restricted to disabled people who experience considerable difficulties in walking. The inability to carry parcels is not a sufficiently good reason in itself.

To be eligible the applicant must either be registered blind, in receipt of the mobility allowance or drive a three-wheeled vehicle supplied by the DHSS. Persons who would fulfill the mobility allowance regulations but are over the age limit may also be issued with an orange badge. The badge is valid for any car providing it is being used by the disabled person, e.g. taxis or friend's cars. Orange badges however will not be issued on grounds of psychological ill health. The disabled person's GP has to complete a medical certificate and a charge for the badge is made. Application forms are available through the local social services office.

Further reading

British Association of Occupational Therapists, *Occupational Therapists Reference Book*, Parke Sutton Publishing, 1986.

Chartered Society of Physiotherapy, *Handling The Handicapped*, Cambridge: Woodhead–Faulkner (3rd edition), 1980.

Department of Transport, *Door to Door – A guide to Transport for Disabled People*, HMSO, 1982.

Patricia A. Downie and Pat Kennedy, *Lifting, Handling and Helping Patients*, London: Faber & Faber, 1981.

S. Goldsmith, *Designing for the Disabled*, RIBA Publications Ltd (3rd edition), 1976.

Philippa Harpin, *With a Little Help. Volume VI Mobility*, The Muscular Dystrophy Group of Great Britain, 1981.

Oxford Health Authority, *Equipment for the Disabled. Walking Aids* (1st edition), 1985. *Hoists and Lifts* (1st edition), 1985. *Wheelchairs* (5th edition), 1982. *Outdoor Transport* (5th edition), 1982.

Ann Turner, *The Practice of Occupational Therapy. An introduction to the Treatment of Physical Dysfunction*, Churchill Livingstone, 1981.

The Ins and Outs of Car Choice, available from DOE and DTP Publications Sales Unit, Building 1, Victoria Road, South Ruislip, Middlesex HA4 0NZ.

Useful addresses

Banstead Place Mobility Centre, Banstead Place, Park Road, Banstead, Surrey SM7 3EE. Tel. Burgh Heath (07373) 56222/51756.

Disablement Income Group Charitable Trust, Attlee House, 28 Commercial Street, London E1 6LR.

Elap Engineering Ltd (car seats), 23 Lynwood Road, Huncoat, Accrington, Lancs. BB5 6LR. Tel. Accrington (0254) 36042.

D. G. Hodge & Son Ltd (car seats), 15 Hurstdene Avenue, Staines, Middlesex TW18 1HZ.

Motability, Boundary House, 91–93 Charterhouse Street, London EC1M 6BT. Tel. 01-261 9644.

Chapter 9

Home assessment and housing adaptations

VALERIE DUDMAN and HILARY SHAW
Community Occupational Therapists, Oxford

The ability to live as normal a life as possible within the home environment is the right of every disabled person. It may be possible to achieve this independence by the provision of small aids and equipment, but it may be necessary for the client and the therapist to consider adapting, altering or extending the existing dwelling. Familiar surroundings, family and neighbourhood support, the accessibility of shops and leisure facilities and possible employment prospects are all important factors which may encourage both the client and the services involved to consider adaptation of his or her present home as the most viable solution rather than considering alternative housing.

A disabled person is not by definition a handicapped person, but this may follow if they are unable to function with maximum independence within the confines of their own home. Many ambulent disabled people are able to use standard facilities even with minimal adaptation, whereas every-day activities may appear to be insurmountable to one who is confined to an unsuitable house with steps, stairs and inaccessible facilities. For those who are wheelchair-dependent special considerations will need to be made – for example, a severely disabled wheelchair user may need to move to a purpose-built dwelling in order to become totally independent.

Layout and general design within the home is an important factor in determining the degree of handicap associated with a disabled person. The decision to adapt the home should only be taken after consideration of the total physical problems, the nature and prognosis of the medical condition, the client's view of his disability, level of handicap and the family situation.

The provision of 'portable' aids or equipment may solve a particular problem but this chapter will be mainly concerned with structural work to the dwelling. Major alterations may include building work or the provision of fixed items such as stairlifts and through-floor lifts. The existing structure of the house need not be altered at all, merely added to or altered internally whilst maintaining the external proportions. Utilising existing space, or changing the use of rooms may well be a more acceptable solution than extending the fabric of the house. It should be noted that although provision for this work comes under the broad responsibilities outlined in the Chronically Sick and Disabled Person's Act and government circulars, the method of execution of these responsibilities may well vary in different areas of the country. It is, therefore, important to identify and thoroughly know individual policies before commencing any major adaptation.

Legislation

It is essential that occupational therapists working in the community should have a clear understanding of the relevant, current legislation appertaining to the provision of services for the disabled. The following legislation described should be regarded as an aid to further reading and not an exhaustive list of all the Acts or joint circulars published. Occupational therapists should ensure that they keep abreast of all new legislation and its implications for their work.

Chronically Sick and Disabled Persons' Act 1970. Section II requires the authorities to provide comprehensive services for the disabled, based on an assessment of their needs, and a fulfilment of those needs where applicable. This includes assistance in obtaining housing adaptations or additional facilities.

Rating (Disabled Persons) Act 1978 – England and Wales only. This Act allows for rate rebates on special facilities provided to meet the needs of the resident disabled person, e.g. additional bathroom, garage or ground-floor bedroom.

Housing Act 1974 (as amended by the Housing Rents and Subsidies Act 1975). Housing authorities were given powers to introduce improvement and intermediate grants to disabled people in the private sector for adaptations required for their welfare, accommodation or employment.

Housing Act 1975. Housing authorities were given powers to carry out adaptations for tenants of public sector housing.

Housing Act 1980. This Act amended the criteria for the provision of grants, i.e. removal of the rateable value limit. Grants were also made available to adapt public sector housing, i.e. tenants could apply individually for consideration.

In 1982 an amendment was made to this Act which led to an increase in the level of grants available for the disabled. The normal rate for the grant became 75% of the eligible expense limit, with a further 90% for the hardship cases. The eligible expense limit was also increased, and has subsequently been increased again to the present limit of £10,200 (1986). London boroughs have a higher limit. (For up-to-date information on current limit levels contact should be made with the Environmental Health Department or Grants Department (Scotland).)

Housing (Scotland) Act 1974 (amended by Housing (Financial Provision) (Scotland) Act 1978). This gives local authorities powers to make improvement grants in respect of houses for disabled occupants.

DOE Joint Circular 59/78, 'Adaptations of Housing for People who are Physically Handicapped.' HMSO 1978. This circular, issued by the Department of the Environment, the Department of Health and Social Security and the Welsh Office, recommended that housing authorities and associations should accept the financial responsibility for structural adaptations to their own housing stock. It did, however, stress that the responsibility for assessing and advising on the housing needs of individual disabled people, including the need for adaptation of their homes, should remain with the social services, in collaboration with health authorities. Non-structural features and the provision of aids and equipment should also be retained by the social services departments (or health authorities as appropriate).

Identifying housing needs

Needs of the disabled person and his or her family

The majority of people who require major adaptations will already be known to the community services. In most cases those who apply directly to their local housing departments, or social services (social work departments in Scotland), will be referred to the community occupational therapist who acts as adviser not only to the disabled person but also to the statutory authorities.

It is important that the needs of the disabled person are recognised early, whether this is by the individual himself, his family, carers, members of the primary health care team or others. There is a fine balance between becoming dependent or achieving and maintaining independence. Conflict of ideas may well occur but must be resolved successfully by discussion and total agreement by all parties otherwise it may lead to dissatisfaction or non-use of the adaptations provided. Ultimately the disabled person is entitled to choose for himself how he lives within the bounds of his disability.

The following three questions need to be answered when identifying the problem.

What is the need –

1. as expressed by the client related to his perception of his disability and role within the family?
2. as identified by the family in which the disabled person functions?
3. as the objective view of the occupational therapist related to medical knowledge, prognosis and nature of the disability?

Possible options

Rehousing. Some disabled people living in the private sector on low incomes, or with low-valued houses, will find that moving to a more suitable property may not be a viable proposition, as the type of accommodation required may not be readily available within their financial resources and the actual cost of moving prohibitive. Even the opportunity to move into purpose-built council or housing association property is not very often possible because of insufficient resources and high demand. However, those living in the public sector do appear to have more of an opportunity to move to more suitable accommodation than those in the private sector. Most housing departments give priority to their tenants who need to transfer for medical reasons and require partially adapted or purpose-built mobility or wheelchair housing.

Adapting present accommodation. It is often possible to improve the use of existing living areas in the home or create more space for the disabled person by very simple measures, e.g. partitioning larger rooms, moving doorways or changing the use of a room. The most common adaptations are ramps, providing showers insteads of baths, downstairs WCs, installing hoists, stairlifts or through-floor lifts.

Extensions to the property. Where there is insufficient space within the dwelling to adapt the property an extension may be the only alternative. Most extensions are built either to the back or side of the house owing to the building line regulations. Factors which will affect this are the position of existing drains, soil pipes, manholes or boundary walls. An extension to the side of a semi-detached house may reduce access to the back garden, driveway or garage, whereas on to the back of a terraced house may cover existing windows which will therefore mean additional light and ventilation being required.

The solution

The identified solution should be discussed with reference to the following points:
(a)   Does it meet all the perceived needs?
(b)   Is the plan feasible, taking into consideration the length of time from inception to completion?
(c)   Will it continue to be suitable in the future?
There may well be more than one solution to the problem, e.g. a stairlift or downstairs WC, but the final deciding factor may be the source of funding and the cost involved.

Funding the project

Both housing and social services departments have limited resources to meet their obligations as outlined in the above Acts. Many have therefore introduced strict criteria for the allocation of these monies and the occupational therapist must know what these are.

The arrangements for funding a project may well be a lengthy process owing to the necessary administrative procedures. Adaptations relying solely on grant aid for finance will often be completed more swiftly than those dependent upon social services for additional funding. Clients should be made aware of this factor to enable them to make an informed decision. Preliminary enquiries about finance should be made at an early stage of the planning to avoid unnecessary delay.

Resources available

Social services departments. Funding may be requested from social services departments in certain circumstances – for example, for those people living on their own, or in privately rented accommodation, who after receiving grant aid are unable to meet the balance of the cost of the building work and related expenses (e.g. architect's fees).

A financial assessment of the client's circumstances will usually be requested to determine the possible level of contribution. Solicitor's fees may also be incurred as a legal document must be drawn up between the social services' solicitor and the client. The social services will usually then act as an agent for the client and be responsible for the completion of the scheme (Fig. 8). Financing may take the form of a grant (e.g. for work under £500) or a long-term loan. A charge is placed on the client's property and certain conditions may be specified regarding payment – e.g. when the handicapped person ceases to live permanently at home or the property is sold.

In privately rented accommodation a direct grant may be payable for work up to a predetermined amount, e.g. £500. However, work costing more than this may only be financed in part, with a maximum level indicated. For example, Oxfordshire social services will finance 50% of the costs outstanding after the provision of an improvement or intermediate Grant up to a maximum of £2000 (1986 levels).

District councils. Many district councils will allocate certain sums of money for adaptations to their own properties. Small

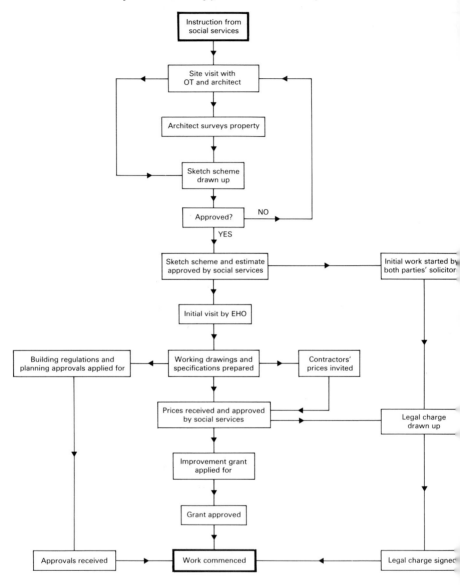

Fig. 8 Flow chart indicating the possible progress of a major adaptation involving social services.

amounts are usually agreed between the occupational therapist and the liaison officer from the council, but larger sums may need approval by a housing committee, or area manager.

District councils may also offer the option of maturity loans for financing adaptation in the private sector, and tenants of the council are also able to apply for an improvement grant, in their own right (Housing Act, 1980).

It may well be important to discuss the implications of adaptations with clients in council housing, who may disentitle themselves from their 'right to buy' by agreeing to adaptations. The 1980 Housing Act states that this right is not present when the dwelling has already been substantially altered to make it suitable for a disabled person. The interpretation of this Act will depend on individual councils and the occupational therapist should therefore be familiar with the current policy operating in the area, and inform the client accordingly.

Home improvement grants. Both improvement and inter-mediate grants are administered by the district councils and London borough councils usually through environmental health officers. Work on a project must not commence before approval for grant aid has been received.

Intermediate grants are mandatory and are given for the provision of a standard amenity. For a disabled person this may mean that the facility is absent or else that the existing amenity is inaccessible to them, by reason of their disability.

Improvement grants are discretionary and are allocated according to the individual council's policy and resources. The Housing Act (1980) removed the rateable value bar which had operated under the Housing Act (1974). Most councils attempt to award between 50% and 75% of the costs, with the possibility of 90% in cases of hardship. All these percentages of costs are limited to the maximum eligible expense limit, as mentioned previously. Generally, the improvement grants are not repayable but the client must undertake to occupy the property for a period of 5 years.

The grant will only be considered after submission of the completed application form, which should include an estimate of costs and detailed plans for the proposed project. Payment of the grant will occur when the work is completed and inspected by the environmental health officer. An agreement is often sought from the occupational therapist to ensure that the completed project does provide for the welfare, accommodation or employment of the client.

In Scotland, adaptations are usually funded by district councils and social work departments. An agreement may have been made between regional and district councils for alterations or adaptations to property in the public sector to be completed by the Confederation of Scottish Local Authorities (COSLA). In the private sector, work is either funded by the social work department, by a grant or by the client, or by a combination of any of the three.

The system of home improvement grants is currently under review, following the publication of the Government's Consultative Document (1985), entitled 'Home Improvement – A New Approach: Government proposals for encouraging the Repair and Improvement of Private Sector Housing in England and Wales', and therefore occupational therapists should be aware of any pending changes.

Housing associations. Funding is available for adaptations to property owned by housing associations and this is detailed in the joint circular of the Department of the Environment, the Department of Health and Social Security and the Welsh Office of 1978.

Charitable funding. This may be considered as an alternative method of paying percentage of the costs not covered by grant aid. However, the sums of money are usually nominal and consequently it will be difficult to raise large amounts from these sources.

Designing for the disabled

The concept of planning and designing for the disabled is not new. There are many books which give general standard measurements recommended for use when designing for the disabled person. However, it cannot be emphasised too strongly that each person is an individual and the effect that illness or handicap will have is determined by his or her abilities, motivation and the environment in which he lives. Any structural alteration should therefore be tailored to meet the individual requirements and based on accurate assessment.

Anthropometric drawings

Anthropometric measurements will enable the therapist to determine the design needs of the client (see Figs 9 and 10). For example, they are especially useful in planning and designing the layout of kitchen facilities, where it is important that careful attention is paid to such items as the positioning of shelves and depths of cupboards.

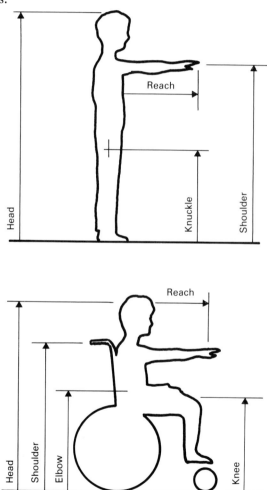

Fig. 9 Anthropometric drawings for ambulant and wheelchair child.

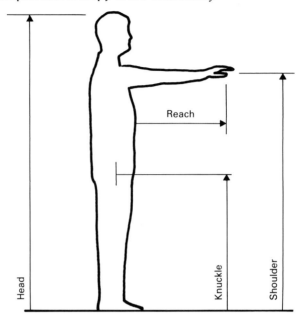

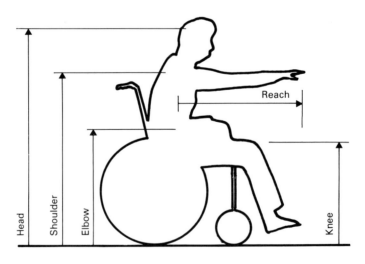

Fig. 10 Anthropometric drawings for ambulant and wheelchair adult.

Scaled plans

The architect will produce drawings of the proposed adaptation with the most commonly used scales being 1 : 20, 1 : 50 and 1 : 100. In order to check that the plans are correct a proper scale rule must be used, so that doorwidths, sizes of rooms and turning spaces are verified. The position of facilities can be determined by positioning scale models of wheelchairs, baths, WCs and showers on the drawings until the most appropriate design is found. This is a more effective method of identifying design options than producing numerous scaled plans (see Figs. 11a and 11b).

Checklists

The occupational therapist should go through a checklist with the architect to determine the specific measurements and equipment necessary which should be carefully recorded. These should include the following:

Type of housing required.
Access requirements.
Kitchen layout.
Bedroom layout.
Bathing/washing facilities.
Floor finishes.
Doors.
Windows.
Refuse systems.
Heating.
Electrics.
Communication aids required.
Leisure facilities.
Specific aids or equipment.

Planning and execution of the scheme

Once a major adaptation has been identified, the work involved in planning and execution of the scheme is similar in both public and private sectors. However, the procedures regarding finance and general administration may vary widely, from both authority to authority, and between sectors.

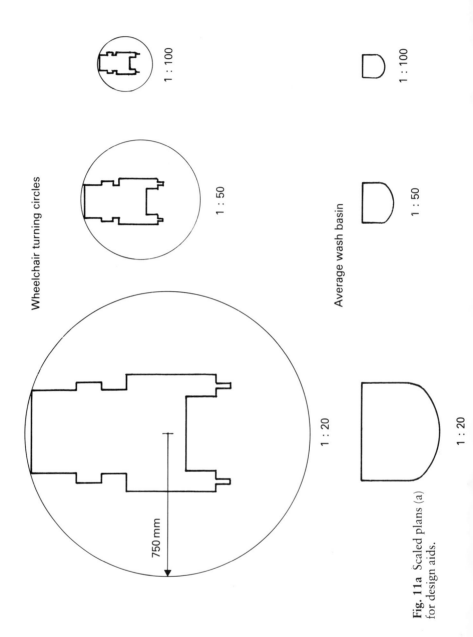

Wheelchair turning circles

Average wash basin

1 : 100

1 : 50

1 : 20

1 : 100

1 : 50

1 : 20

750 mm

Fig. 11a Scaled plans (a) for design aids.

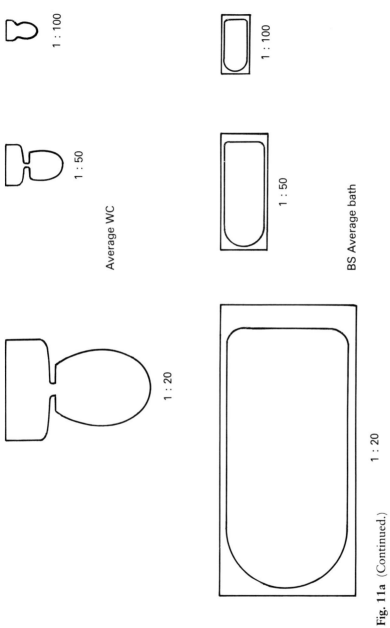

1 : 100

1 : 100

1 : 50

Average WC

1 : 50

BS Average bath

1 : 20

1 : 20

Fig. 11a (Continued.)

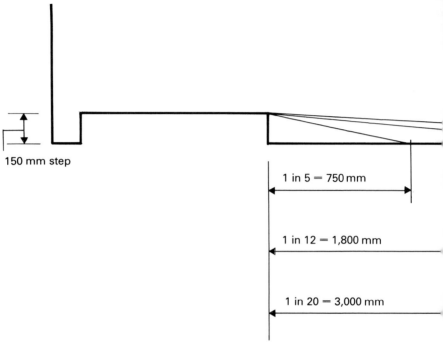

150 mm step

1 in 5 = 750 mm

1 in 12 = 1,800 mm

1 in 20 = 3,000 mm

Fig. 11b Scaled plans (b) for a ramp.

Briefing the architect

A project sheet will help the therapist and architect to keep track of the progress of their work (see Fig. 12).

The following points should be included in discussions with the architect:

1.   The client's disability and needs and present home circumstances.
2.   Details of the proposed work.
3.   Additional equipment/aids to be incorporated into the scheme.

An initial site meeting follows this discussion. A survey of the site will indicate the existing layout and the feasibility of the proposed scheme. The architect will then produce a preliminary sketch scheme based on this survey. Further discussions with the client, occupational therapist and architect will indicate any necessary revisions. A

Ramping gradients (1 : 20)

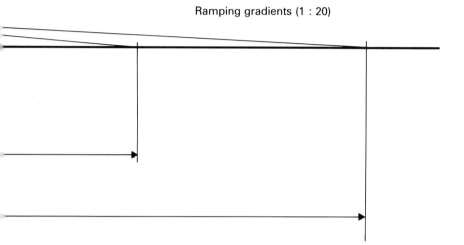

final, mutually agreed sketch scheme can then be produced, with approximate costings, for submission to the funding source for approval. Written agreement should be obtained from the client, indicating his or her agreement to the final scheme to avoid possible misunderstandings at a later date.

Detailed plans and documentation

Detailed plans should indicate the layout of the property to be adapted, and the proposed scheme. The plans may include both ground plans and elevations of the property and should show the present drainage, the electrical points and details of the house construction. Details of the work required will also be shown on the plans, but the types of material to be used, the quality and quantities and method of construction will be prepared as a specification for the builder.

Client's name:
Address:
Occupational therapist involved:
Proposed project:

	Date

Occupational therapist assessment visit
Application completed for agreement to scheme
'In principle' approval received
Brief to architect
Site meeting with architect
Preliminary survey and production of sketch scheme
Acceptance of scheme by all concerned
Visit to site by EHO/grants officer re grant application
Final sketch scheme received (No. noted if necessary)
Final sketch scheme agreed with client
Funding agreed
Funding source
Detailed plans, working drawings received
Detailed plans, working drawings agreed with client
Architect notified of decisions/revisions
Building regulations approval received
Planning approval received
Tenders requested from approved contractors
Selection of contractor
Contract drawn up between client or agent and builder
Legal charge agreed (if appropriate) between client and
    social services
Intermediate/improvement grant application made based on
    accepted tender
Date for commencement of contract
Interim site meeting by architect and/or occupational therapist
Completion of contract
Final check/agreement that work is satisfactory
Completion certificate
Grant paid
Maintenance/defect check — six months after completion
Clearance certificate and payment of final account

Fig. 12 An example of a project sheet used in major adaptations.

The working drawings are used when application is made for planning permission and building regulations approval.

Rules and regulations related to building

Building regulations. The present building regulations (1985) which supersede the 1976 regulations are aimed at ensuring the health and safety of the inhabitants of buildings and any work which involved structural alterations, or extensions to domestic property needing the approval of the building inspector. An example of this would be the provision of a WC and drainage, or putting in a beam when making two rooms into one. There are local water authority bye-laws which govern changes to an existing plumbing system. Apart from fire safety regulations the local authority can relax regulations for special cases. The building inspector will visit the site at various stages in the work to ensure compliance with the regulations.

Planning permission. Internal work is not normally subject to planning permission unless it is a change in use, e.g. dividing a house into flats, but this may still require building regulations agreement. A house extension or garage would require the permission of the planning department, if it exceeds the maximum agreed limit on volume, based on the size of the house. Planning permission is usually also needed in designated conservation areas or for listed buildings. It is always wise to check this point before embarking on any scheme.

Value added tax. VAT is chargeable on all building work – this being introduced in March 1984 at a rate of 15%. The VAT (Handicapped Persons) Order, 1984, subsequently exempted specific items from this charge, e.g. ramps, the widening of doorways and passages, and the installation of a WC and bathroom on the ground floor, specifically for a disabled person. This is only relevant to first-time installations and not to alterations of previously existing facilities (see RADAR *Bulletin* of June 1984).

Estimates and selection of contractor

If the work is being funded and supervised by a district or borough council, or social services, it is likely that the technical services or planning department will hold their own list of 'approved' builders from which they can invite estimates or tenders. Costs are based on the final plan and specifications produced by the architect. In the public sector the work may be completed by a direct labour force, or an outside contractor. In the private sector, where social services are acting as the agent, it is rare for a client to be asked to obtain estimates. Social services will then keep control of the contractor, so devolving responsibility from the client who may have no experience of dealing with this type of task and may find it stressful. Where a disabled person is applying solely for an improvement grant without help from other sources, he or she is normally expected to obtain estimates for the work. In these cases there are several ways of drawing up a list of possible builders; for example,

(a)   contacting local planning departments for advice;
(b)   personal recommendation;
(c)   trade associations;
(d)   local advertisements.

Grant application

Following the preliminary survey and production of a sketch scheme and estimate of cost, the environmental health officer (EHO) will visit the client to explain the procedure for application for a grant, and he will determine which grant is most applicable. Work can only be started on the project after formal approval has been received, although in exceptional circumstances permission may be given to commence before this. The EHO will sometimes visit the site during the contract to ensure that the scheme is progressing satisfactorily, and once the building or alterations are completed, the grant will be paid. It is however possible for the grant to be paid in instalments if necessary.

The contract

Many social services departments produce a standard contract for use in building adaptations. However, for those who intend to work independently the following points will indicate the most important items which need to be included:

1.   The commencement date of the scheme.

2. The completion date with clauses for non-completion or variations in completion dates, with reference to compensation and agreement by the builder to proceed with work on a regular basis.
3. Who will be responsible for obtaining building regulations and planning permission (if appropriate).
4. How alterations to the contract will be agreed.
5. Confirmation that the builder is suitably insured to cover any losses or damages incurred to persons or property during the course of the contract (repair of any defects should be at the builder's own expense).
6. A clear statement of the conditions under which the contract can be terminated by either the client or the builder.
7. The standard of workmanship and materials to be used in the scheme including reference to British Standards and Codes of Practice.

Working with the builder

It is important that all parties have the same well-drawn scale plans and that the builder has clear, written specifications.

It is in the client's best interest to have a formal contract between himself and the builder. This should set out terms and conditions which must be fulfilled as a safeguard against possible difficulties in completing the scheme. The builder must be aware of the problems of the disabled person so that they have daily access to basic facilities such as WC, cooking facilities and a water supply. If this is not possible, this should be identified at an early stage in the planning so that alternative accommodation can be arranged.

The builder may request interim payments during the course of the project, but this should always be agreed prior to commencement of the work and set out in the terms of the Contract. Advance payments may also be requested but this should not be a recommended practice. The contract may, however, state that the client has the right to withhold a percentage of the builder's final account for a period of six months to ensure that the contractor will return to put right any defects which may have occurred during that time.

The actual position of fitments such as wash-hand basins, rails and shower controls, although shown on detailed plans, are often best arranged on site. It is important to keep an accurate record of such

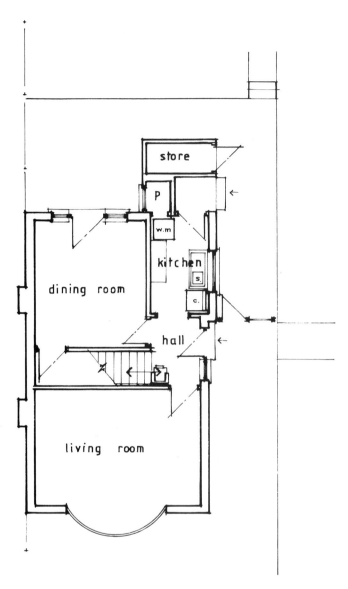

E X I S T I N G

Fig. 13 Plans of Case Study 1.

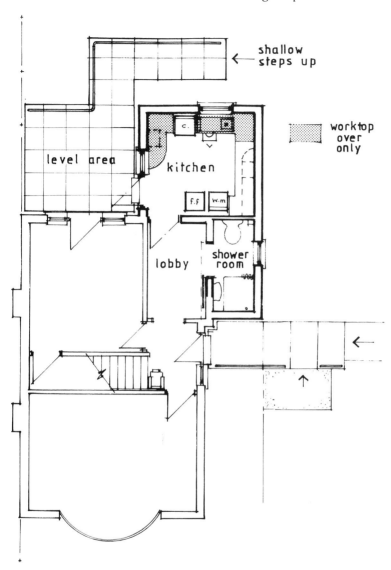

shallow
steps up

worktop
over
only

level area

kitchen

c.

f.f   w.m

lobby

shower
room

PROPOSED

Fig. 13 (Continued.)

meetings and discussions in case of dispute. The builder is usually responsible for arranging the inspection of the site by the building control officer at various stages throughout the project.

Completion of the scheme

A final assessment of the work should be made to satisfy the client, occupational therapist, architect and funding authority to ensure that the project has fulfilled the initial proposals. This may be necessary before finance for the scheme is released.

Case studies

1. This scheme was designed for a 40-year-old woman with severe rheumatoid arthritis affecting all joints which required several joint replacement operations which left her with extremely limited mobility. She lives with her husband in a privately rented house. The existing galley kitchen was inaccessible to her when using her gutter rollator and the upstairs bathroom and WC accessible only by a stairlift. A scheme was therefore drawn up to provide improved kitchen facilities and ground floor toilet and shower (see Fig. 13).

The existing kitchen was used to provide a lobby area to the new 'L'-shaped extension which was designed for both limited ambulatory use with a mobility aid, and wheelchair access. Easy opening drawers, accessible shelves and lever taps were provided.

The floor of the new WC area was covered with anti-slip quarry tiles laid so that part sloped towards a corner gulley, to provide a shower area. The shower controls and a hinged seat were fitted at the appropriate heights and the WC raised by a concrete extension to a height of 24 inches (see Photo. 4).

The scheme was jointly funded by an environmental health grant and the landlords.

2. This adaptation was designed for a 60-year-old man who had suffered eight cerebro-vascular accidents and was now wheelchair dependent. The housing department agreed to rehouse the family as their own home was quite unsuitable and could not be adequately adapted. As some bungalows were in the process of being built, it was possible to make radical alterations to the basic design of one of these for a person in a wheelchair (see Photo. 5).

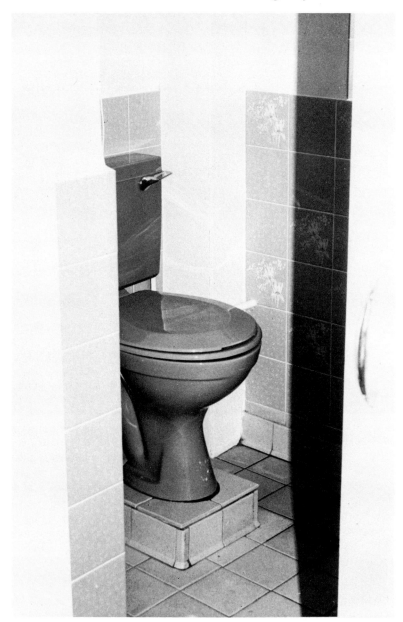

Photo. 4 Case Study 1. Raised WC in new extension.

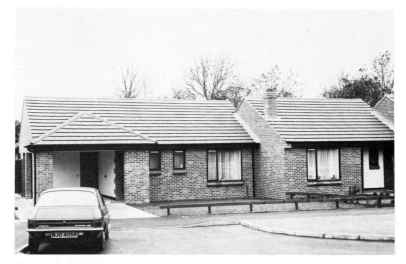

Photo. 5 Case Study 2. The comparison in size of the standard bungalow and the adapted version.

Land at the side of the original plot was used to give maximum circulation space within the bungalow, and to provide a car-port. The kitchen was not altered from the original plan, as his able bodied wife would be mainly using this.

The bathroom (see Photo. 6) was enlarged to allow for equipment and easy transfers and the area at the end of the bath was sloped towards a drainage gulley so that the bathroom had both bath and shower facilities. A sliding door was provided between the main bedroom and the bathroom.

All electrical points, light switches and door handles were sited at a height suitable for operation from a wheelchair.

Level access was provided from the bungalow to the rear garden.

Acknowledgements. We would like to thank Mrs Hilary Grime, Mr Paul Littlefair and Mr Neville Mason for their invaluable assistance in completing this chapter.

Further reading

S. Langton-Lockton and R. Purcell, *Buying or Adapting a House or Flat. A Consumer Guide for Disabled People*, CEH Publication, 1983.

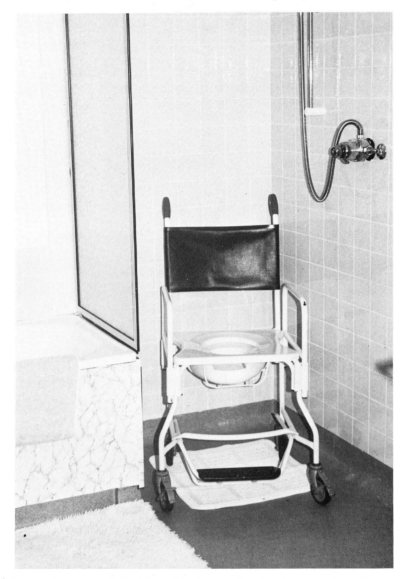

Photo. 6 Case Study 2. Adapted bathroom showing the utilisation of space at the end of the bath to provide a shower area.

Housing Adaptations for Disabled People. The Role of the OT and EHO, CEH Publication.

Cheshire County Council, Department of Architecture, *Made to Measure. Domestic Extensions and Adaptations for Physically Handicapped People*, 1980.

S. Goldsmith, *Mobility Housing*, DOE Publication, 1974.

S. Goldsmith, *Wheelchair Housing*, DOE Publication, 1975.

College of Occupational Therapy, *Resource Book for Community Occupational Therapists*, 1984.

A. Edgington, 'Survey of major adaptations', *BJOT*, Vol. 47, II, 46, 1984.

S. Goldsmith, *Designing for the Disabled*, London: RIBA Publications, 1976.

J. Hunt and L. Hoyes, *Housing the Disabled*, 1980.

Leicester City Council, Planning Department, *Designing for Disabled People*, 1982.

T. Lockart, *Housing Adaptations for Disabled People*, DLF Publication, 1981.

London Borough of Harrow, *Planning for the Disabled*. A Harrow Planning Guide.

J. Penton, *A Handbook of Housing for Disabled People*, London Housing Consortium West Group (2nd edition), 1980.

J. Penton, 'Access for all', *The Architects' Journal*, 16 February 1983.

P. Prescott-Clarke, *Organising Housing Adaptations for Disabled People, Research Study*. London: HMSO, 1982.

University of Edinburgh, Department of Urban Design and Regional Planning, Planning Research Unit, *Planning for Disabled People in the Urban Environment*, RADAR, 1969.

F. Walter, *An Introduction to Domestic Design for the Disabled*. DLF Publication.

DOE Joint Circular 74/74, 'Housing for people who are Physically Handicapped', London: HMSO, 1974.

DOE Joint Circular 92/75 'Wheelchair and Mobility Housing, Standards and costs', London: HMSO, 1975.

DOE Joint Circular 74/78 'Rating (Disabled Persons) Act 1978', London: HMSO, 1978.

Sources

Centre on Environment for the Handicapped, 126 Albert Street, London.

Disabled Living Foundation, 380–384 Harrow Road, London W9 2HU.

Institute of Consumer Ergonomics, Loughborough University, Leicestershire.

Royal Association for Disability and Rehabilitation, 25 Mortimer Street, London.

Scottish Council on Disability, Princes House, 5 Shandwick Place, Edinburgh EH2 4RG.

Wales Council for the Disabled, Caerbragdy Industrial Estate, Bedwas Road, Caerphilly, Mid Glamorgan CF8 3SL.

Chapter 10

The disabled child

JILL RILEY
Paediatric Occupational Therapist, Jenny Lind Unit, Norwich

Although community occupational therapists may only have a few
disabled children on their case-load it is important that they know
the basic principles of treating them and their families. In the space of
one chapter it is not possible to discuss all paediatric medical
conditions, normal child development and applied occupational
therapy and, therefore, basic principles will only be given.

The community occupational therapist must have a basic knowledge of normal child development and of paediatric medical conditions before treating any children. Concentration on the common
occupational therapy areas of work, such as positioning, upper limb
function, activities of daily living and pre-school activities are given
on the assumption that the community occupational therapist is
more likely to come across these needs rather than the more specialised areas of work with which her paediatric colleagues would be
involved. She must first understand the connection between the
paediatric condition and the child's whole development, followed by
the understanding of the parents', care staff's and teachers' role in
the management of the child.

Assessment and treatment

An assessment may be undertaken in the child's home where the
parents can express their needs for the child. Since it is the parents
who are with the child for the majority of the time and responsible
for the child, it is imperative to involve them. Care staff and teachers

should also be brought into any discussions. This will not be completed in a single visit. It will be important to listen to the parents, and others, who are with the child most of the time to find out what are their perceived priority problems and what are their expectations. It will also help to find out whether or not they have a clear understanding of the child's condition; how much they want to 'help' the child in a structured way and the reaction of the other siblings. A school assessment may paint a very different picture of the child from the home assessment – what causes these differences?

The therapist also needs to know what the child thinks and wants for himself. She must also gauge the extent to which she can realistically expect to get co-operation from the parents, care staff and teachers. All are very different and see the child within their own environments. The occupational therapist must use her professional judgement to govern the extent to which she can involve the child in his own treatment programme, and to govern how much the parents, care staff and teachers can be involved. This emphasises again the need for the therapist to be confident in her own knowledge of the subject.

Very few children can be seen once and then discharged. This is not only because of the need for developing a rapport with child and parents, but because of the nature of the rehabilitation required and the fact that children grow and their subsequent needs vary. If the therapist is unable to commit herself to regular and consistent involvement with the family it is better that someone else undertakes the task. All treatment programmes need to be monitored and adapted as the child develops. Special equipment that may need to be provided should be monitored regularly as the child grows and handicaps change. It is easy to visit the school and home once and make a quick judgement thus perhaps raising expectations which are often not realistic. The occupational therapist will only be effective if visits can be maintained in a consistent manner. In some cases what is required more is regular, realistic support with sensible guidelines for the parents concerning the treatment and management of their child for the next ten years or so.

This regular help can be given verbally if the therapist feels that this is the most appropriate method, although some families can cope with written programmes which include diagrams to assist them. It is also possible to record treatment and progress with the parents' participation, for example, Portage,[1] and this can be very helpful to them. Schools, in particular, find written directions helpful. Welfare assistants may appreciate some quite detailed advice for the disabled child in the classroom.

Schooling

The occupational therapist may be involved with children at both special and mainstream schools. Time will be needed to establish relationships with the staff of these and all the principles mentioned above in relation to the parents apply to the school staff. The occupational therapist often finds herself playing a liaison role between the medical team at the hospital and the school. Time will be needed to describe the nature of the child's handicap to the school staff and giving the appropriate advice. She may also need to liaise between the home, school and hospital in order to gain an accurate picture of the child's performance. Such a liaison role puts the therapist in a unique position, especially as her opinion of the child's needs may be requested through the obligations of the Education Act 1981.

The Education Act 1981 promotes the systematic appraisal of the learning difficulties of individual children in consultation with their parents. This takes the form of statementing of children with special educational needs, which is a statutory obligation and may involve the occupational therapist. Assessment is centred on the child rather than on his disability and means the end of the previous classification of pupils by categories of handicap. Section 2 of the Act establishes the principle that all children with special needs must be statemented and, in so far as is possible, are to be educated in an ordinary school and are to be associated with the other children in all the school's activities. The statement gives details of the local education authority's assessment of the child's needs and also specifies the special educational provision to be made for the child, whether in an ordinary or special school. In assessing the child's special educational needs the local educational authority will take into account the views of the parents, and the advice of professional advisers which include the educational, medical and psychological personnel. Parents have the right to see the statement in draft, to offer comments and to discuss it if they wish. Once the school becomes aware that a child has special needs the staff involve the parents and attempt to deal with the situation. This may involve contact with appropriate outside agencies such as occupational therapist, educational psychologists, educational welfare officers, social workers, doctors and other paramedics. If there continues to be concern about the child a formal assessment may follow.

Management

As the occupational therapist's main contribution is towards long-term rehabilitation she is seldom involved in one off treatment sessions. The following describes those paediatric conditions most relevant to occupational therapy:

Cerebal palsy	Arthritic conditions
Spina bifida	Mental handicap
The dystrophies	Head injuries
The multiply handicapped child	Burns and plastic surgery
Children with absent limbs	Perceptuo-motor disorders

The occupational therapist's training in psychiatry and mental handicap gives her a unique role in working with disabled children and their families. There are however areas of work which are more common than others such as:

(a)   *Positioning* – including positioning for rest, play and work.
(b)   *Activities of daily living* – including washing, dressing, feeding, toileting and dressing, transfers.
(c)   *Upper limb function.*
(d)   *Perceptual function.*
(e)   *Communication.*

The therapist must always make a detailed assessment of each child as this will be essential in establishing a baseline and in providing guidelines to treatment. Reviews must be made regularly for treatment to remain effective. The following short guide to assessment provides some treatment aims.[2]

General impression

1.   Parent–child relationship.
2.   What can the child do (abilities) and how?
3.   What can he not do (disabilities) and why?
4.   What does he try to do abnormally and why?

Having established a general impression of the child's functional ability, one may go on in more detail to assess specific problems.

A more detailed physical assessment may then be carried out in conjunction with the physiotherapist. On examination, prior to positioning, the occupational therapist must observe the following:

Postural patterns:
Asymmetries.
Predominant flexor or extensor hypertonus.
Tonus quality at rest and under stimulation.
Contractures present or threatening.

Head control and trunk stability:
In prone position.
Supine, pulled to sitting.
Sitting.

Sitting:
When placed on floor or chair.
Sitting up unaided from floor (may be from floor to chair).
Balance in sitting.

Standing:
Standing supported or holding on to support.
Sitting to standing using hands/without hands.

Positioning

Having understood the nature of the disabled child's medical condition and assessed the child with all concerned, the occupational therapist can commence planning the treatment programme. It is quite probable that the priority will be to provide the child with some form of functional positioning, e.g. a chair which need not only involve sitting. The disabled child needs to alternate his position as much as the able-bodied child. Alternative positions include lying prone, supine, side lying, standing and kneeling.

Aims of seating

1.   Function.
2.   Prevention of deformity.
Good positioning is not necessarily achieved by expensive seating

materials. It is only achieved by understanding the nature of the child's movement disorder, the major disorders being cerebral palsy, spina bifida and the dystrophies. There are spastic, athetoid, ataxic and hypotonic types of cerebral palsy as well as many different forms of neural-tube defect and neuromuscular diseases, which makes it inappropriate and undesirable to give a list of chairs and positions for specific handicaps. Every child is different and every child changes in his positioning requirements. The only principles therefore are to:

(a)   understand the movement disorder;
(b)   review the position regularly;
(c)   alternate the position;
(d)   ensure that those handling the child know how to position him properly in the equipment.

In general however the optimum sitting position is as shown in Fig. 14.

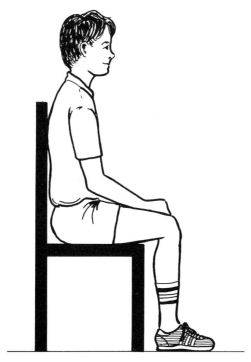

Fig. 14 Ideal sitting position.

The back should be well supported, hips at right angles, knees flexed at right angles and the feet well supported. This can only be obtained by starting at the pelvis and fixing it, and then working out from there, otherwise the child's whole body will not be stabilised (Fig. 15).

Following an assessment the disabled child may fit into one of the following categories:

(a)   predominantly flexor pattern;
(b)   predominantly extensor pattern;
(c)   predominantly hypotonic;
(d)   with athetoid or ataxic movements.

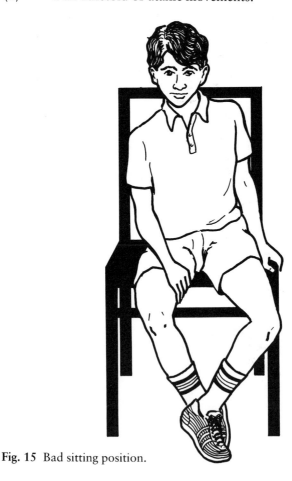

Fig. 15 Bad sitting position.

However, they may of course display a combination of these either symmetrically or asymmetrically.

The general rule of fixating the pelvis applies to all of these categories. They must not be permitted to 'swim' around in their chair otherwise the two aims of positioning, that is, function and prevention of deformity, will not be achieved.

One of the main deformities to be prevented is the 'windswept hip', or the asymmetric hip deformity in cerebral palsy.[3] The aim here is to abduct the 'adducted' hip and to maintain neutral or external rotation. This of course can only be done if the pelvis is correct and stable. The following table suggests points to look for when seating the disabled child.

Type of movement disorder	*Seat modifications*
1. Predominantly flexor pattern Aim for:	
(a) Symmetry	Foot rest In extension at hips
(b) Extension	Harness High table/tray
(c) Adduction/abduction of hips according to asymmetry	Grab bars Pommel Adduction/abduction pads
2. Predominantly extensor pattern Aim for:	
(a) Symmetry	In flexion at hips Protracted shoulders
(b) Flexion	Floor-runners Grab bars
(c) Lean forward	Possibly 'soft' foot rest Possibly short back/head rest
(d) Adduction/abduction of hips according to asymmetry	Pommel Adduction/abduction pads
3. Predominantly hypotonic Aim for:	
(a) Symmetry	Slight extension of hips Back rest with head rest

(b) Support   Arm support
                                          Trunk support
                                          Harness
                                          High table/tray
                                          Foot rest
                                          Grab bars

4. With athetoid or ataxic movements
Aim for:
(a) Symmetry   Grab bars
(b) Stabilisation and fixation

Chairs may be obtained commercially; a visit to a specialist paediatric centre[4] would be useful before purchasing any seats; or the occupational therapist could make the chair herself. Obviously it is ideal if they can be adjustable.

Custom-made seats are also available commercially in the form of moulded and matrix seating. Again, a visit to a specialist paediatric centre to learn about these materials will prove helpful. Both matrix and moulded seats can be attached to wheelchairs, however the artificial limb and appliance centre have to approve the prescription of both of these in wheelchairs provided by the Ministry. Both matrix and moulded seats can also be supplied attached to major or baby buggy chassis. It is of course possible to adapt the wheelchair seating position with appropriate cushions, harnesses, pommels, trunk supports, head supports, seat angles and trays in the same way as one adapts a free-standing chair.

Other equipment is available for alternative positions such as the following:
>   *Prone* – wedge and prone board.
>   *Supine* – wedge.
>   *Side-lying* – side-lying board.
>   *Standing* – standing frame.
>   *Kneeling* – standing frame.
>   *Mobility* – hand-propelled tricycles and trolleys.

The same principles apply here as to seating. It is imperative for the occupational therapist to understand the nature of the child's movement disorder and to fully acquaint herself with the piece of equipment before placing a child in it. Again a visit to a specialist paediatric centre would be helpful here.

Activities of daily living

Positioning principles apply to dressing, feeding, washing and toileting. Having established the optimum functional position for the disabled child this position must be maintained as far as is possible in activities of daily living. In dressing, for example, the child may be helped by sitting on the same chair/position in which he works. He may even need to have a table nearby where he can lay out his clothes in a correct sequence orientation for his needs, and a footstool may also be needed. Grab rails like those on the child's chair may be useful in other parts of the house, for example beside the toilet, to help give stability and to aid independent transfer. A grab rod for the ataxic or athetoid child on his tray may help in stabilising one arm and hence the shoulder girdle in readiness to feed himself (see Fig. 16). It is also important to carry the ideal position over to bathtime when the disabled child can be both playing and learning at the same time.

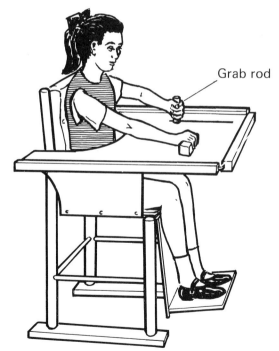

Grab rod

Fig. 16 Sitting using a tray and grab rod.

The following information provides a useful checklist for activities of daily living.

1. *Dressing*
Child's attitude.
Position dressed; position dresses self.
Garments taken off; garments put on.
Techniques used.
Aids used.

2. *Toilet*
Child's attitude.
Indicates need.
Routine.
How does he get to toilet?
Position for pulling down clothes.
Getting off toilet?
Position for pulling up clothes.
Aids required.
Techniques used.

3. *Bath*
Child's attitude.
Routine.
Access to bath.
Washing routine.
Play.
Out of bath.
Drying position.
Aids required.
Techniques used.

4. *Feeding*
Child's attitude.
Routine.
Position for feeding.
Drinking.
Utensils.
Aids required.
Feeding pattern:
   tongue thrust
   gagging

continuous sucking
inability to close mouth
swallowing
Types of food:
liquids (hot and cold)
crisp
raw
slippery
chewy
large bites and chew

5. *Other positions*
Bed.
Sleeping pattern.
Car seat.
Mobility buggy/wheelchair.
Play/nursery/school.

Many aids are available commercially, but they must be comfortable and practical and achieve something for the child otherwise they will not be used. Aids to daily living provide a practical solution to many of the disabled child's functional difficulties, but they must be prescribed by a therapist who knows about the child, his disability and his family. These aids do not only provide practical help but they can also provide a focus for the family on which:
(a)   to pinpoint many anxieties
(b)   the family can place hope for a 'cure'.
Caution must therefore be taken before prescribing them.

There are also various techniques based on treatment methods which require specialised training; for example, neurodevelopmental treatment (Bobath)[2] and conductive education (Peto).[5] Such techniques can be used in feeding and dressing as well as gross motor therapy.

Upper limb function

Having positioned the child he is then ready to use his hands. This applies to activities of daily living, play and work. Assuming that they are motivated and that distractions are at a minimum, the child's upper limb function should develop. However, further assessment may be necessary. For example:

(a)   Is the child seeing and hearing properly?

(b)   Is the table at the correct height?

(c)   Is the table too far away?

(d)   Is the material being presented from the correct side?

(e)   Do the upper limbs themselves require special attention?

(f)   Is the material/activity/instruction appropriate for the child?

(g)   Does the child have a perceptual problem?

In studying normal development the occupational therapist learns how gross and fine movements develop side by side, and how the normal child gains perfect hand eye control by the time he reaches school age. The hand is an important sensory organ, an initiator of action and a means of communication. However, many disabled children have been denied such experiences and their upper limb may require special attention. This is particularly true of the child with cerebral palsy. A normal baby's hands are held and played with, and using his reflex grasp the baby will catch hold of and be pulled into a sitting position. He may grasp a rattle, inadvertently touch his mother's face with an open hand, and in consequence the eye hand control begins and so does the bonding between mother and child. The normal baby develops and begins to explore his environment and his own body but the cerebral palsy baby, for example, is deprived of these experiences. Consequently occupational therapy may aim to familiarise the child with his own hands. The assessment must include observations of the child's hand function in all positions: supine, prone, sitting and standing. The assessment should include the following:

1.   Does the child have a grasp reflex? Dominant/non-dominant hand?

2.   Does the child have an asymmetrical tonic neck reflex? Left/right? Does he fist the hand to the extended side?

3.   Can the child bring his hands in front of his face? Left/right? How does he do it?

4.   Can the child grasp? Left/right/both together? Can he release his grasp? Left/right/both together? In what position? How long can he hold the grasp? When does he let go (movement of head, noise, etc)?

5.   Can he make hoops with his fingers? 1–2, 1–3, 1–4, 1–5? Left/right/both hands? In what position?

6.   Can the child put his hands down at the side? In supine

position; sitting on a table; kneeling; sitting grasping on a chair or stick in front? Does he know what it means by stretching elbows?

7.   Is the startle reflex present?

8.   Are his hands weak, hypermobile joints in fingers?

9.   Is the thumb hidden in the palm? Left/right/both hands? In what position?[6]

Other areas that need attention to develop upper limb function include training for midline orientation. It is much better for the child to hold his head in midline as this helps focusing and attention. Holding an object, in a side lying position using both hands and then moving the object from and towards the face, is a starting point for developing a controlled grasp. This can be slowly made more difficult until it can be done in varying positions. Having grasped an object and held it still, the child must learn to release in a controlled fashion. Activities can be planned working with sticks using finger rhymes to promote the finer movements of the hand. Gross motor exercises can also be used.

Any upper limb training must be done not in isolation but as part of the total picture of the child in light of his total movement disorder.

Pre-school assessment

To establish whether the instructions and the equipment are appropriate for the child, a further assessment must be carried out. This assessment should give a baseline on which to plot the child's pre-school skills. A standardised pre-school assessment may be used covering such areas as body image, drawing skills, laterality, threading, eye hand co-ordination, use of scissors, block building, ball-throwing, colours, shapes, sizes, shape constancy object/picture recognition, position in space, spatial relationships, figure ground, copying block design and stereognosis.[7]

It is of course essential that such tests are standardised. Having established a baseline, the areas which are not age appropriate become apparent and so the treatment programme begins.

The Frostig test referred to above is the Marianne Frostig test of visual perception which establishes a child's level of performance in each of the five areas of visual perception.

1.   Hand eye co-ordination.

2.   Shape constancy.
3.   Position in space.
4.   Figure ground.
5.   Spatial relationships.

The current edition of this test was standardised on more than 2,100 children and is thus a very useful one for establishing the baseline and giving guidelines for treatment.

Some children with severe disabilities involving the upper limbs may be prescribed typewriters. This tends to be more appropriate for the older child. However, if the child suffers from severe ataxia or muscular weakness it is often useful to start them typing early on. Various models are available with special adaptations, such as condensed or expanded keyboards and key guards. Many of these adaptations can also be applied to computer keyboards. Word processors may also be appropriate. Typing skills have to be taught but the ability and speed of learning will partly depend on the comfort of the child's position and whether or not they are at their most functional position. POSSUM adaptations are also available for children.

Other communication aids fall into the province of the speech therapist as well as the occupational therapist, such as pointer boards, which can be operated by a variety of switches.

There will be other aspects that the occupational therapist will need to consider as the child grows including support to the parents through many uncertainties and apprehensions so that the child does not become smothered but is allowed to develop and explore the world around him and become part of it.

References

1. Portage Association, King Alfred's College, Sparkford Road, Winchester, Hants.
2. Bobath – The Bobath Centre, 5 Netherall Gardens, London NW3 5RN.
3. D. R. Scrutton, 'Seating for asymmetric hip deformity in non ambulant multiply handicapped children', *Orthopaedic Engineering*, 1978.
4. Child Development Centres: The Wolfson Centre, Institute of Child Health, Mecklenburgh Square, London WC1; The Newcomen Centre, Guy's Hospital, St Thomas' Street, London SE1.
5. Peto Conductive Education, Ingfield Manor School, Five Oaks, Billingshurst, Sussex RH14 9AX.
6. E. Cotton, *The Hand as a Guide to Learning.*

7. M. Frostig, *The Frostig Programme for the Development of Visual Perception*, NFER – Nelson Publishing Co.

Further reading

Development

J. H. de Haas, Mrak van Blankenstein, Ursula R. Welbergen, *The Development of the Infant*, William Heinemann Medical Books, 1975.

Mary Sheridan, *Children's Developmental Progress from Birth to Five Years* and *Spontaneous Play in Childhood from Birth to Six Years*, NFER Publishing Co.

Paediatric conditions

E. M. Andersen and B. Spain, *The Child with Spina Bifida*, London: Methuen, 1977.

Barbara M. Ansell, *Rheumatic Disorders in Childhood*, London: Butterworths, 1980.

Association for Spina Bifida and Hydrocephalus Publications, Tavistock House North, Tavistock Square, London.

Berta and Karel Bobath, *Motor Development in the Different Types of Cerebral Palsy*, London: William Heinemann Medical Books, 1978.

Daniel Boon, *Cerebral Palsy*, Indianapolis: Bobbs-Merrill Company Inc.

Steven V. Fisher and Phala A. Helm, *Comprehensive Rehabilitation of Burns*, Baltimore/London: Williams & Wilkins, 1984.

Sophie Levitt (Ed.), *Children with Brittle Bones* and *Paediatric Developmental Therapy* (Chapter 13), Oxford: Blackwell Scientific, 1984.

Muscular Dystrophy Group of Great Britain Publications, Nattrass House, 35 Macaulay Road, London SW4 0QP; Tel. 01-720 8055.

A. Richardson and A. Wisbech, *I Can Use My Hands*, Toy Library Association, Seebrook House, Darkes Lane, Potters Bar, Herts EN6 2HL.

E. Robertson, *Rehabilitation of Arm Amputees and Limb Deficient Children*, London: Baillière Tindall, 1978.

Spastics Society Publications, 12 Park Crescent, London W1N 4E4; Tel. 01-636 5020.

Treatment

Nancie R. Finnie, *Handling the Young Cerebral Palsy Child at Home*, William Heinemann Medical Books, London, 1974.

M. Frostig, *The Frostig Programme for Development of Visual Perception*, NFER – Nelson Publishing Co, 1966.

N. Gordon and I. McKinley, *Helping Clumsy Children*, Churchill Livingstone.

Sophie Levitt (Ed.), *Paediatric Developmental Therapy*, Oxford: Blackwell Scientific, 1984.

Sophie Levitt, *Treatment of Cerebral Palsy and Motor Delay*, Oxford: Blackwell Scientific, 1982.

Muscular Dystrophy Group of Great Britain, *With a Little Help*

L. Routlidge, *Only Child's Play*, William Heinemann, 1978.

Phillipa Russell, *The Wheelchair Child*, Human Horizons Series, 1978.

Useful addresses

The Bobath Centre, 5 Netherall Gardens, London NW3 5RN.

Child Development Centres – The Wolfson Centre, Institute of Child Health, Mecklenburgh Square, London WC1; and The Newcomen Centre, Guy's Hospital, St Thomas' Street, London SE1.

Peto, Conductive Education, Ingfield Manor School, Five Oaks, Billingshurst, Sussex RH14 9AX.

Chapter 11

The management of the severely disabled and the terminally ill person

SHEILA PARSONS
Occupational Therapist, Caroline House, Norwich

'It is not what a man has lost but what he has left that is important'.[1]

Disabled people are living in a changing environment as the emphasis is moving from residential to community care. The benefits of these changes will be very important for large numbers of the disabled population by giving them independence, choice and responsibility, perhaps for the first time in their lives.

At present many *severely disabled people* are living in residential institutions – either national health or social service units or private homes such as those as provided by the Sue Ryder or the Leonard Cheshire Foundations. They all vary in their approach towards their residents, but the majority have a philosophy of 'care' rather than 'independence'. Consequently the residents often become completely dependent for all aspects of life.

Difficulties arise as the expected lifespan becomes longer due to improved medical knowledge and the care received in the protected environment of residential homes. With good dietary control, warmth and personal care, the general health of the residents remains high and the chest infections which can cause demise in many neurological conditions are less frequently seen. Consequently the number of beds available becomes fewer, preventing the admission of those whose disability is such that residential care would normally be advised. However, others are deciding that they do not wish to remain in the restricting environs of an institution and are wanting to live in the community.

The transition to community care, together with increased provision of day centres and social amenities, means that integration with the well population will gradually take place. There will, however, still be a need for beds for those who are so disabled that home, family and other carers can no longer provide the required care.

Ideally the individual should be allowed the choice of where and what type of accommodation he or she would like to make their home, but with the present shortage of specialised accommodation this is not always possible. However, every person must be consulted and included in the decision making affecting their future.

The *terminally ill* are included in this changing outlook. Previously most terminally ill people were cared for in their own homes, and often died in pain and discomfort. Hospitals were unable to admit them owing to insufficient beds as, until recently, they were more able to provide for those with a chance of recovery. General practitioners and district nurses were the mainstay of community care and provided all possible help. Now with the development of the hospice movement and increased experience in the use of analgesic drugs the outlook has changed. People in the closing stages of life are helped and cared for by professionals who are able to provide symptom relief and who are trained to ease the anxieties felt at this time by patients and relatives. There is an atmosphere of cheerful, relaxed peace in these units and dying is accomplished with dignity and calm. The bereaved are also cared for and receive support for as long as required. This type of care is now being carried into the community with specially trained hospice staff, who provide the support to enable the patient to remain in his own home. Gradually hospice philosophy is also changing, as more people are admitted for shorter periods for symptom control and relief before returning home and, perhaps, continuing attendance as out-patients for day care.

Severe disabilities can be divided into three broad categories, as follows.

1.   Congenital disability, including disability acquired in early childhood.
2.   Acquired disability, through trauma in teenage or adult life.
3.   Progressive disability through disease.

The mental state of the individual is affected in different ways depending on how the disability was acquired.

Congenital or early onset disability may cause the least mental agony for the sufferer. Children are very accepting and are usually capable of overcoming the most severe handicap. What they have not known they do not seem to miss. Youngsters find their own way to do things and accept help as a means to an end without embarrassment or loss of self esteem.

Disability acquired through trauma is of very sudden onset and hospitalisation is required. Shock is deep and the full realisation of the extent of injury takes time to be absorbed. The mental state may resemble that of a bereaved person, going through the stages of shock, denial, anger, bargaining and depression before acceptance and hope is attained. This can take several years and cause great stress within the family. A young person may feel he has lost all the normal expectations of youth with job prospects drastically changed. Some disabled young people reject their former friends, unable to reconcile themselves to their disability and it can take a long while to form new relationships. Marriage prospects may seem to disappear and all point of life lost. Bodily functions take on a new and horrendous importance, causing social embarrassment.

Relatives can find this a very difficult period. Parents have their own grief to cope with and may find it difficult to support their offspring. They may need to face the prospect of caring for an invalid just when they were looking forward to a freer, more restful period of life. Consequently, relationships may change and collapse under these pressures. Therefore, when dealing with these people it is important to remember that the whole family needs special consideration and allowances must be made for tensions that appear.

With *progressive disability* the person is often unaware of the prognosis of the disease and time is needed to accept each new problem as it arises. The realisation that they can no longer take an active role in raising their children or support the family financially can be hard to accept. A greater burden is placed on the healthy partner which increases as the disability progresses. In many cases this leads to a breakdown in relationships. Sometimes, of course, the opposite happens with great new strengths being found. Where brain damage occurs the resulting increased disability is most distressing for the family.

In all these groups there will be those who will go through the remainder of their lives with a chip on their shoulder and feelings of aggression towards society. These people need special understanding, although it may prove impossible to help them very much. The occupational therapist must accept failures with the successes and help them as much as is allowed.

Special needs

In helping severely disabled people it is important to remember they have the same basic social and psychological needs as everyone else, such as the following.

1.   The need to belong.
2.   The need to be recognised as persons in their own right.
3.   The need to be given opportunities to pursue ambitions and to develop interests and skills to enable them to progress in life.
4.   The need for security. To feel 'safe' in themselves and their surroundings; and also for financial independence and security.
5.   The need to have faith in themselves and in those helping and to know that people also have faith in them.
6.   The need to make their own mistakes and to be responsible for them.

There are also special needs to enable the disabled person to live in the community. These are related to physical, psychological, emotional and work needs.

Physical needs

In order to remain in the community, assessments for the usual aids for personal care will be needed, but it is important to take into consideration those who may be using them, such as family, carers, volunteers or paid help. If a person wishes to live alone any outside help needed should be organised before discharge and a good rapport established with these helpers. They will need to be included in the rehabilitation programme so as to be aware of future responsibilities and to gain confidence in the use of equipment.

Environmental control systems can give some measure of independence and choice within immediate suroundings. There are some very sophisticated systems available which may be controlled by voice, slight head movement or blinking an eye.

Transport for the disabled is improving. The range of outdoor vehicles is very wide and some can be driven from a wheelchair. These obviate the need for constant transfers and provide an important advancement in independence.[2]

Psychological needs

Mental stimulation is necessary for maintaining health, preventing depression and for achieving an optimistic outlook. Most centres of higher education provide facilities for the disabled and many towns run courses for hobbies. Attendance at a class, club or day centre not only provides stimulation but opportunities for creating new relationships, interest and outlooks (see also Chapters 17 and 18).

It is important to give the disabled person the security of knowing that help will be available if problems arise. They may come from any members of the care team, someone who has a good rapport with the family and who can communicate through the right channels to obtain the help needed.

When there is a relentless downhill course as in motor neurone disease, efforts need to be made to ensure some quality of life right to the end. For example, one gentleman who knew he was dying spent his last week thus – Monday, shopping all afternoon; Tuesday, typing; Wednesday, he attended a football match; Thursday, he saw his children; and on Friday he died. Although a very exceptional man, it is good to know that such quality of life is achievable.

Where people are experiencing difficulties in coming to terms with their disability and cannot decide what they want from the future, a clinical psychologist may be able to help identify motivating factors and provide a strategy for personal reconstruction.

Emotional needs

Counselling may be an ongoing process to enable people to cope with increasing disability and the knowledge that fewer parts of the body will function normally. It may also be a help in dealing with family problems. If arguments develop between the parents, the whole family begins to distintegrate. Emergency admission for short-term care may help in these situations whilst the care team consider a more appropriate regime to ease the situation still further.

Problems may arise with the young disabled in coming to terms with emotional situations involved with maturing physically but being unable to develop as a normal youngster with members of the opposite sex. Encouragement should be given for activities involving able-bodied young people to allow relationships to develop. They will be better able to cope if a certain amount of risk taking is acknowledged and accepted.

Difficulties may occur with the physical side of married life and it may be wise to seek advice from those qualified to deal with such problems.[3]

Employment needs

With high unemployment figures work is becoming more of a problem for disabled people. A limited amount of home work is available, but this is usually very poorly paid and does not provide the stimulus of contact with workmates. Sheltered workshops and day centres are able to provide some light employment, but again pay is poor and the work is often repetitive (see Chapter 17).

Functional assessment

Functional assessments provide a useful means of introducing and maintaining independent living.

Congenital disability. Functional assessment with these youngsters is an ongoing process as the child grows and becomes heavier for the parents to handle or as he wishes to lead a more independent life. Parents often ask for help as the need arises but care should be taken to keep in touch with those families who do not do this.

When school leaving time approaches the future must be considered. Schools help with career advisers but assessment for living alone will be needed for those progressing to college or university. Confidence in basic life skills may need boosting (see also Chapter 17).

Acquired disability. Maximum independence should be achieved prior to assessment for life in the community. With practice and increasing confidence it is often possible to discard aids initially provided for this purpose. Many will depend on electrical equipment for hobbies or work and it is essential to ensure that an adequate number of suitably positioned electrical outlets are installed. When considering hobbies, clubs providing similar interests should be investigated. These present a good medium for integrating with the able bodied and of making new friendships. Most libraries have extensive lists of such organisations in the area.

Progressive disability and terminal illness. All the foregoing considerations will be salient for people in this group, but more input by the occupational therapist will become necessary as the disability increases. Careful follow-up and reviews will be needed with aids to assist the carer and for the comfort of the patient.

Wheelchairs will probably need to be changed with, maybe, more support pads to prevent slipping and to achieve a more comfortable position, as well as allowing varying positions for different activities. Sheepskin panels available from artificial limb and appliance centres can relieve pressure on the back and seat. Cushions need regular checking as the average life of most is only about two years. However good the cushion is, long periods sitting in one position will produce discomfort. Providing a different cushion for morning and afternoon use may help the situation. Padding arm rests and covering them with cotton material helps to prevent pressure sores on elbows and forearms.

It is essential to be familiar with several methods of transfer with different applications. Lifting people with cancer can be very painful for them, so it may be advisable to introduce a hoist at an early stage.[4] Many patients and carers find the progression to wheelchairs and then to using a hoist very traumatic and introducing the idea of an aid to be considered when problems become too great can set people thinking and prepare for acceptance. A hoist is often more readily accepted when the patient falls to the ground and the carer is unable to pick him up. For this reason it may be appropriate to commence teaching him to use the hoist with the patient on the floor, so that its real use can be quickly appreciated. Adequate teaching in their use is essential to carers if accidents are to be avoided. Hoists, however, need regular checking for metal fatigue (cracks) as these too have a limited life.

Many people find shower or sanichairs very uncomfortable;

however, this can sometimes be relieved by padding the backrest and seat. Foam is not good as it takes a long time to dry and is often cold and damp when next used. An alternative is bubble plastic, such as the large, strong type used for camping mattresses. This easily cuts to size and is simple to fix.

For patients in bed who find it difficult to sit up, a bed elevator may be helpful. These fit under the top of the mattress and are elevated by air pressure which is controlled by the patient.

Talking books, music, environmental controls and sufficient visitors all help to maintain morale and prevent boredom. The ability to call for help is important, especially when there are difficulties with speech. Environmental controls usually have a built-in alarm, but if these are not available another system must be sought. A whistle on a flexitube and placed within reaching distance may help, or it may be possible to attach an air switch to a bell which can be positioned to use any remaining movement, e.g. under the chin, between the knees or under the head. In these difficult late stages of a disease, admission to a residential setting or hospital may need to be considered, to help both the patient and the carer. This is often more readily accepted if intermittent care has been part of the regular pattern.

With the gradual increase in the number of day centres attached to hospitals, hospices or younger disabled units ongo' ıg assessments and symptom control can be more easily achieved without full admission. Problems that are just beginning can be noticed and appropriate action taken. This is especially important in the care of patients with rapidly deteriorating conditions. Aids need to be thought of in advance so that they are available when required. This means that the therapist must think ahead all the time.

There is now a very good Motor Neurone Disease Association which, in common with many other similar societies, produces leaflets of use to both the patient, the family and the professional.[5]

Special equipment used in the care of severely disabled

1. *Wheelchairs.*   See Chapter 8.
2. *Armchairs.*   A range of chairs is available on the market. Some are made to measure and can have casters for manoeuvrability. Chairs need to be low enough for the feet to reach the floor, but not so low as to make transferring

difficult. Cushioning and support need careful assessment for long-term comfort.

3. *Hoists.*   As some older types of hoists have a very wide base the width of doorways need to be checked. The quickfit type of sling is best for the severely disabled as no lifting is required.

4. *Mobile arm supports.*   Available from artificial limb and appliance centres, and issued to people using wheelchairs. Assessments take time and can be complicated, therefore, their benefits must be proved to the patient for them to be accepted.

5. *Environmental controls.*   Hugh Steeper and Possum controls are available from the Department of Health and Social Security. Others, such as the Popstar typewriter, have provision for some environmental controls and an alarm. With modern technology, controls are available to enable most disabled people to use aids in assisting independence. However, DHSS aids can take several months to be installed from the initial request.

6. *Typewriters.*   Many portable electric typewriters are available, and prices have become more reasonable. Keyboard guards are made for some models.

7. *Reading aids.*   Large print books are available through local libraries and some now hold stocks of books on tape. Talking books are provided for the blind and talking newspapers are often produced locally and delivered free. There are numerous page turners but the choice depends on the type of book to be read, as some will not take paperbacks and magazines. Very few page turners are produced for newspapers, but Quest Education Designs have a very good one for tabloid newspapers.

8. *Communication aids.*   The use of these depends very much on the physical dexterity of the patient and several different ones may need to be tried. Machines that also have a printout are often preferred as they can be used by those unable to use a typewriter.

With the rapid change in technology new aids are constantly appearing. Information on the latest developments may be obtained from the Disabled Living Foundation or by contacting the local joint aids or communication aids centres.[6,7]

Aids library

The need for such a library is obvious when expensive aids are required for assessment, or short-term loan, at short notice. Such aids include page turners, magnifiers, special cushions, chairs, limb support machines, environmental controls and communication aids. The library can be used by occupational therapists, speech therapists or others. It is important that sufficient quantities of each aid are available so that long waiting periods are eliminated. Equipment can be loaned for short periods, perhaps whilst awaiting delivery of their own aid, or to those who will probably only need the equipment for a short period of time because of their deteriorating condition. Funding for such a library can be obtained from joint finance and charities.

Communication needs

Where speech is affected by disease, communication is one of the most frustrating problems for the severely disabled. Trying to make oneself understood is exhausting. While some manual dexterity remains, communication can be achieved by pencil and paper, or by the use of a communication aid. Alphabet boards are useful while the patient is still able to point, however vaguely, towards a letter or word. Boards can be made with the letters spaced to suit the user and to include words he or she uses often. Finally, when all else fails, an eyeboard may help (see Fig. 17). The patient looking up, down or

A B C	D E F	G H I
J K L	M N O	P Q R
S T U	V W X	Y Z

Fig. 17 An eyeboard.

level indicates the line he wants, then, looking left, right or straight ahead, indicates the square. This leaves three letters to select from. This method is slow, but quicker than going through the whole alphabet. Some people can indicate 'yes' or 'no' with eyebrows or shutting/openings the eyes. All questions must be formed for yes/no answers. Sometimes it is easier to communicate through a person familiar with the patient, who can interpret for him. This saves much misunderstanding and is less tiring for the disabled person.

Case studies

1. Cedric aged 25 years

Cedric fell backwards whilst playing football at school and sustained a tetraplegia at C5/6 level. After one year of treatment he was independent, with aids, for feeding, washing, shaving, typing, writing and propelling his wheelchair. While awaiting rehousing into a purpose-built bungalow with his parents, Cedric remained in a younger disabled unit. He found it difficult to accept disability and rejected all his former friends, was introverted and unwilling to consider retraining for work. He refused to go outdoors in his wheelchair. After 18 months in the unit, the bungalow was ready, but Cedric would only visit it occasionally and would not allow his family to care for him.

During this time his typing had progressed to a high standard and some outwork had been completed. He also attended the District General Hospital to encourage outings, new relationships and for occupational therapy. He completed several woodwork projects although no progress with regard to employment was made.

He improved socially and became friendly with a nurse who cared for him in his bungalow. He was thus discharged from the unit, but still attended for out-patient physiotherapy. After holidaying with his girl friend they decided to buy a home of their own. Cedric still did not wish for employment although he was interested in computers and completed an economics course. A trust fund set up after the accident helped financially. After a further four years Cedric's girl friend became pregnant and they were married. In due course a son was delivered.

Conclusion. Following many initial difficulties Cedric was able to accept his condition and now enjoys a full life as a husband and a father. This demonstrates how long acceptance of the disability can take and how it is sometimes necessary to begin an entirely new life.

2.   *Erica aged 28 years*

After a diagnosis of multiple sclerosis was made, Erica became divorced and returned to live with her parents, taking her two-year-old son with her. Deterioration was rapid with very few remissions and after five years she was unable to walk, had marked tremor in upper limbs and head and her speech was almost unintelligible.

A garage was enlarged and made into a self-contained unit for Erica (see Fig. 18). Her eyesight deteriorated and though she could still use her possum typewriter from memory she was unable to read or watch television. She had talking books and music, but relied on her father for all aspects of care, whilst her mother cared for her child. Erica was upset by the fact that her son hardly knew her as his mother. It was suggested that she got some children's books on tape and made a special period each day for listening together. This helped for a while, but as Erica's memory began to fail she was unable to remember people, facts or how she spent her time. She received intermittent care in the younger disabled unit to help her parents and at present is spending two weeks out of every six in the unit. She also receives weekly outpatient physiotherapy, and as problems occur they are dealt with by an occupational therapist. She enjoys her visits to the unit and partakes in social activities there, but is unable to remember them for long. Her son is now seven and regards his grandparents as his parents.

Conclusion. This young woman's condition was exacerbated by her pregnancy. Her parents, who were looking forward to retirement, now face increasing work in her care and in the upbringing of their grandson. The time will soon come when Erica will need permanent residential care as her father is finding the task increasingly difficult, but the care of her son will continue for years to come.

References

1. Inscription on the wall of the Philippine Cheshire Home.
2. The Nippi Scooter. Special Vehicle Designs Ltd, Ravenston Road, Industrial Estate, Coalville, Leicestershire LE6 2NB
3. The Sexual Problems of the Disabled Group, 49 Victoria Street, London SW1.

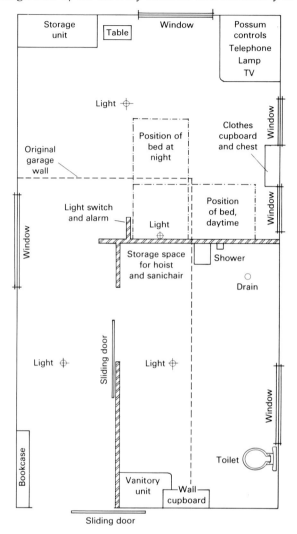

Covered way to house

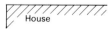

Fig. 18 Plan of garage alteration and extension for Erica.

4. *Handling the Handicapped – a guide to lifting and movement of disabled people.* Chartered Society of Physiotherapists. Cambridge: Wood-head–Faulkner Ltd. (2nd edition) 1980.
5. Motor Neurone Disease Association. Secretary Mrs E. A. Gretton, 7 Lorimer Road, Gedling, Notts.
6. *Equipment for the Disabled*, Mary Marlborough Lodge, Nuffield Orthopaedic Centre, Oxford.
7. *Occupational Therapy Reference Book 1986*, British Association of Occupational Therapy.

Further reading

Freda Clarke, *Hospital at Home, the alternative to general hospital admission*, Macmillan, 1984
Graham Hurley, *Lucky Break*, Milestone Publications, 1983.
Ann Shearer, *Living Independently*, Centre on Environment for the Handicapped and King Edwards Hospital Fund for London, 1982.
Christine Tarling, *Hoists and their Use*, Heinemann, 1980.
Margaret and Jack Wymer, *Another Door Opens*, Human Horizon Series, Souvenir Press, 1980.

Chapter 12

The needs of elderly people

ANNE DUMMETT
District Occupational Therapist, Islington Health Authority

The philosophy of geriatric medicine and care of the elderly person cannot be encompassed in one simple definition for it is very wide ranging. However, there is an absorbing range of diagnostic and remedial opportunities that exist with old people. Enormous rewards can be reaped from the unexpected recovery after critical illness, in the successful management of protracted disabilities, or in assuring comfort and dignity in their last hours. People who survive to a 'ripe old age' do so more through their own genetic make-up combined with the fundamentals of survival – warmth, food, fluids and companionship.

Few old people ask for help unless they feel really ill, if their mobility has created a significant loss of independence, or if they become so handicapped that outside support is essential for ordinary standards of hygiene and self-care to be maintained. Invariably the problem is that the elderly person, or relative, waits too long to ask.

The occupational therapist has the opportunity of using the widest variety of skills with the elderly. The pace may be slower than working with other groups, but there is scope and opportunity for assessment and problem-solving in a truly multi-disciplinary environment.

Specific medical problems of which to be aware

Cerebro-vascular disease

'A stroke is an acute disturbance of cerebral function of presumed vascular origin with disability lasting more than 24 hours'.[1] A stroke is only one of four main presentations of cerebro-vascular disease. The others are transient ischaemic episodes, disorders of postural fixation and balance, and dementia. Acute cerebro-vascular accidents (CVAs) are covered in detail in medical textbooks but some points are emphasised here as follows.

1.   At least 20% of patients with CVA have ischaemic heart disease as well.

2.   About 7% of cerebral tumours present as hemiplegia of sudden onsets but strokes attributable to vascular disease can appear gradually with headaches.

3.   Stroke patients are at risk of hypothermia because the onset is often early in the morning and the patient may lie uncovered for several hours after collapsing before being found.

Points of management to be remembered

(a)   The elderly person cannot be expected to have a better mental or physical level of activity after a stroke than before it. It is essential therefore to have an estimate of former capacity.

(b)   No two hemiplegias are alike and thus any rehabilitation programme must be flexible and designed to meet the individual's needs.

(c)   Emphasis must be on remaining ability rather than disability as the tendency of many people who have suffered a stroke is to bemoan their losses.

(d)   Failure to progress indicates that it is important to develop a sensitive index highlighting causes of delayed recovery, – i.e. problem orientated medical records (POMR).

A systematic assessment is essential to

i.   determine the person's progress;

ii.   assess the person's needs and design an appropriate programme;

iii.   act as an index to effectiveness of treatment of the individual.

Mental barriers to recovery and response

1.   Inability to learn through
    (a) clouded consciousness;
    (b) aphasia;

(c) memory defect;
(d) dementia.

2.   Disturbed perception through
     (a) anosognosia
     (b) neglect of hemiplegic side;
     (c) denial of illness or paralysis;
     (d) disordered spatial orientation;

3.   Disordered integrative action.

4.   Disturbed emotion.

A hemiplegic person seldom has insight to complain about these mental barriers, and it is usually an observant relative or neighbour who notices incongruous behaviour.

Faints and falls—control of posture, difficulty in walking

Balance exercise and constant practise are essential to encourage the best use of compensatory movements in the elderly after illness. However, no person can do better than their peak of activity before the illness.

Elderly people often complain of difficulty in walking. Disorders of gait fall into three principle groups:

1.   Those attributable to 'old age', i.e. a shortened step, or loss of awareness of the vertical stance.

2.   Those accompanied by uni- or bilateral cortico-spinal lesions.

3.   Those related to peripheral neuromuscular disease.

Faints. Old people use a variety of terms to describe transient disturbances of conciousness, such as 'attack', 'weakness'. They are also often embarrassed by their frequent 'attacks'/'accidents' and may be reluctant to volunteer information about them. Possible causes for these may include

(a)   simple faints through stress, heat or pain;
(b)   postural hypotension, i.e. on standing up too quicky;
(c)   carotid-sinus syndrome;
(d)   epilepsy.

Falls. It is thought that women are far more liable to falls than men, and that the incidence of these increases steadily with age in identical proportion to both sexes. Falls are easily classified according to intrinsic or extrinsic causes. Underlying most falls there appears to be an age-related defect in the control of posture and gait. Old people may *trip* and *fall* owing to senility, parkinsonism ataxic or apraxic disorders of gait; or to impaired eyesight, visual inattention, or domestic hazards such as loose carpets, ill-lit stairways or loose wires. They may *stumble* because of clumsiness resulting from a physical disability such as arthritis. They may *sway* owing to deteriorating control of balance, or to vertigo caused by postural hypotension, adverse drug reaction or vertebral basilar inefficiency. Elderly people may suddenly *collapse* due to cardiac syncope.

Drop attacks. These are instantaneous falls occurring most commonly in women without warning or loss of consciousness. These are usually as a result of brain stem ischaemia and there is immediate recovery of function. The elderly usually recognise their failing but realise there is little they can do about it other than avoid sudden movements and protect themselves from environmental hazards. Help can be given by advice on proper clothing and domestic aids, e.g. good lighting, handrails, uncluttered rooms, well placed furniture and floors without loose mats and clutter, or even highly polished floors.

Parkinsonism

Incidence in the over-sixties in the United Kingdom is 15 per 1000. In older people it occurs in association with cerebro-vascular disease and phenotinazine intoxication. This disease follows a slow, unremitting course downhill towards total dependency. Old people often complain about slowing down, a sense of weakness, tremor or stiffness, that it is all too easy to dismiss incipient Parkinsonism simply as 'old age'.

Old people do not have a dramatic response to medication and although there may be a marked improvement in rigidity and bradykinesia the elderly person may still be heavily handicapped through loss of normal postural fixation, unpractised righting reflexes, weakness of disused muscles and loss in confidence. A programme of rehabilitation should include, in particular,

(a)   postural and balance exercises in front of a mirror;

(b)   practise in turning in bed; getting in/out of a chair (raised to appropriate individual height if necessary);
(c)   walking exercises;
(d)   washing, bathing and dressing practice.

In Parkinsonism associated with arterio-sclerosis, the instance of dementia is high and mental deterioration limits the possibility of re-education owing to impaired grasp, concentration and memory.

Late-onset diabetes

Age and obesity are the outstanding factors predisposing diabetes mellitus. Most, when first diagnosed, are well over the age of 50 years and the incidence increases with each decade over this age. The onset is sometimes as sudden and severe as in youth, but more often it is gradual and less dramatic.

Elderly diabetics can be divided into three groups:
(a)   Those whose hypoglycaemia can be controlled by diet.
(b)   Those who need insulin.
(c)   Those who respond to anti-diabetic drugs.

Accidental hypothermia

This has been recognised in Great Britain as a specialised hazard of old age. The endogenous causes for hypothermia are as follows:
(a)   Those directly related to old age such as impaired temperature regulation, infirmity and immobility, slowness.
(b)   Malnutrition.
(c)   Illness.
(d)   Reaction to drugs.

Mortality is high and therefore prevention is better than cure. Constant surveillance of old people at risk, provision of warm clothing and bedding, safe heating appliances and encouragement to activity are a few methods of helping to prevent this.

Incontinence, pressure sores

Incontinence is a symptom and not a disease (see Chapter 13). Pressure sores are either superficial or deep. Some ageing shins are more prone to break down than others and when the elderly person is for instance malnourished, thin, or on steroid therapy this is more true. Vigilance, careful handling, and observation can prevent these superficial abrasions. Deep pressure sores are predisposed by:

(a)   lowered tissue vitality;

(b)   impaired peripheral circulation;

(c)   sensory and motor deficits preventing mobility.

Prevention is far better than cure for all sores and acute awareness of susceptibility is critical. This is determined by general condition, mental state, physical capacity and incontinence.

Malnutrition

Old age leads to physical and mental infirmity, social isolation or deprivation of one kind or another. Malnutrition is usually the consequence, *not* the cause, of such disorders as dementia or depression. Advanced signs are listlessness, hypothermia, pallor, slow pulse, low blood pressure and oedema. It is important to try to encourage old people to take the trouble to maintain a balanced diet and ensure that they are able to cook and prepare food with appropriate aids such as a food blender, small microwave oven and built up cutlery.

Multiple pathology and loss of senses

In old age both precise diagnosis as a basis of treatment and the assessment of disability are often compromised by a number of active or inactive pathological processes affecting the outcome. Degenerative and locomotor disorders are pre-eminent in the elderly. The outstanding limitations are imposed by cardiovascular disease, restricted exercise tolerance in ischaemic heart disease, transient cerebral ischaemia, postural imbalance and strokes, intermittent claudication, gangrene and amputations due to peripheral vascular occlusion, arthritis, neuro-muscular disorders, cancer and the tendency to resistant pulmonary infections and thrombo-embolism. Common respiratory diseases resulting from the ageing process are pulmonary thrombosis, carcinoma of the bronchus, pulmonary embolism, concurrent respiratory disease and failure.

Growing old automatically affects the locomotor system, resulting in loss of physical strength, reduced range of movement, stooping, and loss of height. The senses are also affected, resulting in reduced vision, hearing, smell and taste. These systems/senses will be affected to a varying degree but there will also be a continuous decline.

Social problems and loneliness

Many elderly people become labelled 'social problem' as a matter of course. However, solutions often present themselves when the problems are assessed and analysed. As one grows older one generally experiences the need for a more restricted, but deeper, intimacy. Invariably those now old and alone will find boredom, fear and loneliness an increasing and very real factor. Under these circumstances regression, passivity and withdrawal crowd in. Frequent causes of becoming a social problem and/or lonely are as a result of

(a)   anti-social behaviour, i.e. unacceptable eating habits;

(b)   poor self-care and hygiene;

(c)   loss of hearing or sight which lead to isolation, withdrawal and unresponsiveness (often resulting in the label 'demented' or 'confused');

(d)   bereavement through the loss of spouse, friend, pet or familiar surroundings.

Re-locating an elderly person will set up a chain of reactions; they may well become confused, disorientated and appear unresponsive. However, with a little forethought it is possible to overcome to a degree, if not wholly, these problems. Elderly people must be treated with respect and dignity. Wherever possible the person who knows the individual best – perhaps the community occupational therapist or geriatric visitor – should visit the elderly person to help them adjust to the difficult transposition. Any information regarding the person is useful, remembering that an elderly person will not change well-worn habits.

If aggression, paranoia or withdrawal are apparent, rather than automatically labelling the individual, the therapist should analyse the situation, review the information acquired and consult the individual. For example, the reason for 'incontinence' should be questioned for it maybe that judicious positioning of a bed or commode will enable someone with limited mobility to reach the toilet or aid in time. Review of the total situation and the elderly individual is essential.

In this competitive society elderly people, particularly the very old, express a great fear of going out, and of being rejected by the young because they feel 'crabby', 'wrinkled', 'slow', and 'uninteresting'. Fear is generated also because they feel particularly vunerable to abuse and attack. These fears result in the old staying indoors – alone.

Through an appropriately designed programme, and with previous careful assessment, specific group and individual treatment to help overcome these problems can be applied. For instance, individual counselling and discussion regarding a specific bereavement or fear will enable the older person to become more objective as well as less isolated. Group activities such as a quiz on the highway code with pictures of the appropriate symbols, a cookery group related to the season, and self-help activities, e.g. what to do/not to do when a stranger comes to the door, will establish self-confidence, retain memory and sensory patterns and provide social interaction. Instead of evading an expressed or discovered problem it is important that the occupational therapist devises a means, or activity, to reach a solution. For example, unhygienic home surroundings which have resulted in an elderly person being labelled 'a social problem', unable to carry out self-care hygienic activities and being admitted to hospital with a multitude of problems could have a very simple solution. A home visit in such a case revealed that due to the flushing mechanism of the toilet being extremely stiff, likewise the sink taps, it was impossible to flush the toilet or wash anything. This elderly, immobile woman had resorted to using any receptable, had become confused, withdrawn, lost all self-respect and malnourished through her own self-degradation. Simple and careful re-organisation of her home situation, continual occupational therapy and physiotherapy at the day hospital, designed to meet her specific needs, facilitated progress and she could return home psychologically and physically refreshed.

Group activities for the elderly should encompass well-known tasks and stimulate the senses, as well as being designed to stimulate social contact, physical activity, induce confidence and reinforce independence (see Photo. 7).

There is a great variety of aids on the market, enabling elderly people to remain at home with greater confidence and independence. For instance, communication devices to the front door so that keys need not be left in the latch or dangling from a piece of string can be installed (see Photo. 8). Such aids enable the identity and business of the visitor to be ascertained before the door is opened – thus preventing, to a great extent, unsolicited visitors, and making the elderly person feel more secure.

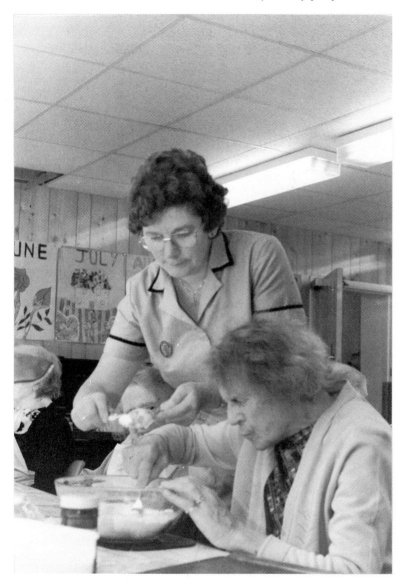

Photo. 7 Cookery sessions stimulate innate skills and form a useful social activity.

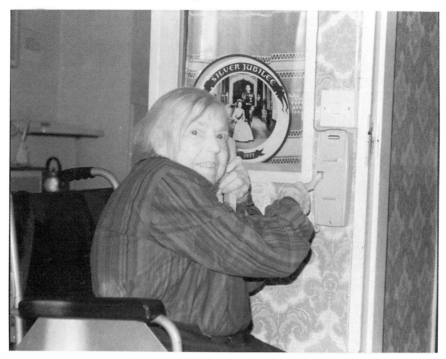

Photo. 8 An automatic door-opening system.

Functional assessment

The occupational therapist in the multidisciplinary setting is able to indicate how well, and at what level of independence, an older person can manage – whether he or she can return/stay at home, will require help from social services, e.g. in the form of meals on wheels or home help, because they cannot manage the more complex tasks of shopping and cooking, or require constant support.

The occupational therapist carries out an assessment to ascertain the nature and extent of the problems (see Fig. 19). A programme is established and, to be effective, must be modified, reviewed and re-assessed frequently as the individual progresses and improves. The programme must concentrate on personal, physical, psychological, social and domestic needs, i.e. exercise tolerance, motivation, mental capacity, motor and sensory deficits, and postural control, the aim being to restore the individual to maximum ability. The complexity of social, psychological and physical factors contribute to the following areas:

1. Personal independence.
2. Domestic skills.
3. Mobility.
4. Social and leisure activities.

Whatever the prognosis, personal independence, confidence and harmony are paramount. Using a specific assessment form (one example is illustrated in Fig. 19) acts as an aide memoire. However, all the activities must *actually* be assessed before any accurate comments can be made. It is not good enough to accept verbal responses, and the recording should be exact, i.e. 'Mrs E. can walk 50 yards with frame and no physical assistance'; rather than 'Mrs E. can walk with frame independently'. The latter enlightens no one as to the true capacity of Mrs E., who may as a consequence be placed in a situation unsuitable to her capabilities – e.g. home.

In order to help establish the level of cerebral function a test can be carried out, and repeated regularly (see Fig. 20). The outcomes of this test facilitate programme planning and, in part, defines how confused a person is. An elderly person labelled 'senile dement' or 'confused' may prove to be 'confused' due to the fact that he or she is in a different environment and this test will etablish this over a period of time. Once the elderly person has adapted and settled she will function at her usual accustomed level.

Maintaining independence

The occupational therapist may well be, and should endeavour to be, involved in ensuring that the environment fosters independence. For instance, the therapist may advise on appropriate furniture, wheelchairs, special equipment and heights of rails. If a family understands the elderly relative's capabilities and has been instructed by the therapist in the ways in which to provide help, then maximum co-operation and harmony interfamilia is likely to be achieved. An awareness of how they can best help themselves should be included in this education, i.e. avoiding back strain through correct use of bath aids.

On admission to any unfamiliar environment well-established patterns of behaviour are disturbed. This can affect body functions, sometimes contributing to incontinence and constipation. Disturb-

Functional assessment			
Name	Rating scale	1. = Totally independent.	3. = Needs assistance.
Record no. ...... Date		2. = Independent with aids.	4. = Totally dependent.

1. Mobility Walking – on own – with aid Wheelchair Stairs Car Public transport Transfers Bed – on – off Chair – on – off Bath – in – out Toilet – on – off 2. Clothing Undressing – lower – upper Dressing – lower – upper Fastenings Zip Buttons Velcro Socks/stockings Shoes Splint 3. Self care Washing Bathing Toilet Make-up Shaving Hair 4. Eating and drinking Knife and fork Fork Spoon Cutting food Cup/glass		5. Cooking Lifting saucepan Filling kettle Vegetable preparation Opening jars Opening tins Make and pour tea Meal – 1 course – 2 courses Washing up Drying up Shopping 6. Household Housework – light – heavy Laundry Ironing 7. Safety Cooker – gas – electric Hob – light – use Grill – light – use Heating – turn on – turn off 8. Communication Dysphasia Aphasia Able to read Able to write Use telephone Handle money 9. Mental and physical state Orientation Memory Attitude Mood Hearing	Vision Balance Co-ordination (rate as good–poor, 1–4) 10. General activities Use of keys Lights Pick up self from floor Pick up objects Bolt and unbolt door Open and close windows Strike match Manage a meter Open and close cupboards 11. Children Feed Wash Dress Pushchair Transport 12. Home situation (tick as appropriate) House – private – council Flat – private – council Part III home Lives – alone – with family – with friends – others	

Fig. 19 A functional assessment form.

Simple tests of cerebral function	

Name .... Age .... Ward........
Date of admission .... Right- or left-handed.............
Date test performed .... Time ....
Observer's name...

Tests	Score
Memory	
1. Name.	2 1 0
2. Age.	2 1 0
3. Address or last address before admission. (Q. Where did you live before you came into hospital?)	2 1 0
4. Ask patient to remember address – enquire after 10 minutes exactly.	5 4 3 2 1 0
Vocabulary	
5. Define the meaning of: ship, **fabric**, remorse, reluctant, sanctuary.	5 4 3 2 1 0
Calculation	
6. Subtract 17½p from 50p.	2 – 0
Orientation	
7. State time of day (morning, afternoon or evening).	1 0
8. State whereabouts (room or hospital).	1 0
Speech	
9. Name objects on a tray. Five should be held up separately – coin, button, pencil, key and scissors.	5 4 3 2 1 0
10. Obey simple commands e.g. 'Put out your tongue'.	1 0
11. Read simple instructions e.g. 'Raise your arms'. Can instructions be obeyed?	1 0
12. Read aloud.	1 0
13. Write name spontaneously.	1 0
Practical tests	
14. Copy patterns with right hand using three matchsticks.	1 0
15. Copy patterns with left hand using three matchsticks.	1 0
16. Copy patterns with right hand using five matchsticks.	1 0
17. Copy patterns with left hand using five matchsticks.	1 0
Toy tests	
18. Posting box.	6 5 4 3 2 1 0
19. Pyramid rings.	6 – 4 – 2 – 0
Check answer to memory test (question 4).	
Total score	☐

To score: circle the appropriate figure under the 'score' column, according to the patient's ability to get the answer, or parts of the answer, right. Add up the score at the end.

Fig. 20 A cerebral function test.

ance of sleeping and eating patterns may increase confusion, and may indeed lead to frustration and aggressive behaviour (as mentioned before). Any intervening personnel should work together to achieve a basic level of independence so that essential tasks as moving about in bed, walking or wheeling to the toilet/bathroom, dressing and feeding, can be performed. The occupational therapist as she develops a rapport with the elderly person, must get to know the pace at which tasks can be achieved and share this vital information with others. It is important that the individual is allowed enough time to master difficult tasks and thus build up his self respect and confidence, e.g. dressing with simple appropriate usable aids if necessary.

In many instances the therapist will need to advise the relatives and other relevant people on methods by which tasks are most easily achieved as a result of functional assessments, programmes, reviews and conclusions. A specific programme may be devised in conjunction with others, i.e. community speech or physiotherapist, or local authority home staff, to overcome particular problems. For instance, when a person with a stroke becomes absorbed in a creative activity familiar expressive speech may be used which is not used during a formal speech therapy session; or the taking of an elderly person into a local authority home for a social activity can alleviate the fear and apprehension of such an institution.

Each elderly person makes social contact in a different manner. He may want to be able to listen and talk to others, feel useful, or just be left alone. Through the earlier devised programme a situation is created in which the elderly are encouraged to gain confidence and self-esteem. Aids can help with leisure, hobbies, and interests, e.g. wooden card holders. Attendance at a day centre, luncheon club, adult education centre or local club helps to maintain social contacts for the individual. Regular day care provided by some homes, offering a hot meal, company and a change of environment gives the opportunities for regular communication to be maintained with those at risk.

Of the increasing number of elderly people, the majority do not go into care, but remain in their own home. The complications likely to occur with ageing have already been mentioned, e.g. loss of balance, which is frequently made worse by incorrect heights of chairs, toilet or bed, and by little or nothing to hold on to for stability. Many small aids and adaptations will enable the elderly person to retain his independence and reduce risk. For example, a bed downstairs to eliminate the danger of a bad fall on the stairs and correctly positioned and secured furniture at the right heights. There are resources within access which provide the necessary support, supervision, rehabilitation and social contacts such as day centres, day hospitals, local clubs and adult education or recreation centres.

For those elderly people unable to look after themselves at home any longer a residential home may be the only reasonable alternative. Wherever possible, advice should be given on appropriate aids and adaptations and the individual's pace and abilities must be handed on to the staff in the 'home'. Some community occupational therapists are involved with the teams allocating residential places. In addition they work with the staff in homes developing activity programmes aimed at increasing and maintaining independence of the residents, or providing mentally and physically stimulating activities.

Housing managers and occupational therapists

In some boroughs occupational therapists work very successfully with housing managers to ensure that, through their knowledge of an individual's capabilities, special housing is properly allocated. This sometimes includes the occupational therapists working closely with the architects on designing appropriate housing for the disabled elderly.

Elderly people are referred to continuing care only as a final resort when they are unable to become or maintain sufficient independence, in spite of assessment, treatment, review and support. A critical element of the therapist's role is to become involved in activity programmes which provide intellectual stimulation and encourage mobility and physical activity. Creative projects (such as the one illustrated in Photo. 7) will be devised to enable those with varying handicaps to make a valid contribution. There is endless scope for using creative and educative media, for taking part in social activities, gardening and outings. Volunteers, relatives, handcraft teachers and others can all be involved to help provide these activities and encourage maximum participaton and stimulation.

The intervention of the occupational therapist in the rehabilitation of the elderly in various settings does not necessarily lead to dramatic results, but affords rich rewards in the responses and progress achieved as well as being a decisive element in maintaining or developing the self confidence, independence and esteem of an elderly person.

References

1. George F. Adams, *Essentials of Geriatric Medicine*, Oxford University Press, 1981.

Further reading

J. A. M. Gray and H. McKenzie *Take Care of Your Elderly Relative*, Allen and Unwin, 1980.
O. L. Jackson, *Physical Therapy of the Geriatric*, Churchill Livingstone, 1983.
P. M. Cornish, *Activities for the Frail*, Winslow Press, 1983.
Lorna Rimmer, *Reality Orientation*, Winslow Press, 1983.
M. W. Shaw, *The Challenge of Ageing*, Churchill Livingstone, 1983.

Chapter 13

Incontinence

JUDITH HARLE
Continence Adviser, Stockport Health Authority

Incontinence is not an illness, but a symptom of a medical condition. Nobody dies from incontinence, it is not life threatening and it is often dismissed lightly by doctors and nurses as part of growing old and therefore, inevitable – or it is only to be expected in women who have had children! Too often these prevalent attitudes lead professionals and sufferers to believe that nothing can be done to help. Incontinence is a hidden problem and much time, energy and money are spent in an attempt to hide the fact, even from their nearest and dearest, rather than trying to solve the problem.

Who suffers?

Incontinence is a widespread problem which affects all age groups and classes. How much of a problem it is depends upon an individual's personality, and knowledge. Present-day research is showing that obstetric practices in the past, or an individual's lifelong habit of straining at stool may well have helped cause the incontinence by weakening the pelvic floor. Research is starting to produce statistics which indicate some of the causes of incontinence, and also shows where prevention should be practised. One of these studies, looking into the prevalence of urinary incontinence,[1] shows that less than one third of those claiming to be incontinent received any help; that more women were affected than men (see Table 3), and that childbirth increased the risk of incontinence.

A second survey into the prevalence of faecal or double incon-

Table 3 Incidence of incontinence.

Already known to health and social service agencies			Postal survey, i.e. not known to any agency		
Age	*15–64*	*65+*	*15–64*	*65+*	
Men	0.1%	1.3%	1.6%	6.9%	
Women	0.2%	2.5%	8.5%	11.6%	

The figures are as a percentage of the population as a whole.

tinence[2] showed that very few of those affected in the community received any help or advice. Although the estimates of the prevalence are tentative, they did show that the incidence in the population as a whole was twice that known to health and social service agencies.

Both of these surveys indicate that the numbers of those affected by incontinence was far higher than had been thought.

In 1983, £36 million was spent by the health service on incontinence aids, and an estimated 3 million people are thought to be incontinent.[3] We must therefore be looking to the future by promoting continence or managing incontinence in such a way that people can ask for help openly and expect to receive it. This utopia is far from with us, especially under present financial constraints.

How do people suffer?

Incontinence causes much suffering even though the person may not be ill.

Physically this is easy to see. The skin may be sore and red. The sufferer may be very tired indeed, especially if the problem is one of frequency and urgency particularly through the night so that sleep is badly disturbed. If in addition there is extra linen to be laundered, additional energy is required to tackle this task, which many find difficult, leading to much distress and sometimes depression. Carers too become extremely tired.

Psychologically and emotionally. Depression can be an actual illness brought about by incontinence and together these may cause isolation. People are acutely aware that they and their homes may smell, wet patches may be left behind, or clothing may be stained. The shame felt is so great that there may well be a denial that there is a problem. Worry about finances may also lead to depression as the cost of providing pads, pants; washing and drying linen; and replacing ruined clothing and furnishings is a great burden. Pads cost around £2.75 for twenty from chemists, and may only last two or three days.

Frictions within families can occur because of the consequences of the incontinence. There may be denial on the one hand, and a complete lack of understanding on the other. One attitude that is often seen is that the person who is incontinent is lazy, whereas others believe that they have to put up with incontinence because they are growing old. All of these factors create a vicious circle, and both sides of the family may require skilled counselling to come to terms with the situation.

Socially. Incontinent people tend to isolate themselves, and gradually stop going into public places or shopping, for fear that they may have an accident. They stop inviting people to their homes or visiting the family in case someone finds out. Many lose a sense of their own worth as a person and end up with their only contact being the milkman from whom many elderly people receive the staples of life.

People are reluctant to seek help because of the enormous social taboo which there is surrounding the elimination of the body wastes. We do not talk about it, and there are many expressions which are used to avoid saying that one is going to the lavatory. A child is taught that there is a right time and place to empty his bladder, and that it should be done in private and that it is rude to talk about it. This teaching is carried through to adult life and it is a shameful thing for anyone to admit that he has not got full control over his bladder, and to lose control over his bowel is even worse. People are made to feel outcasts if they transgress against this unwritten rule.

The role of the continence adviser

As health authorities realise the importance of promoting continence, continence advisers are being appointed. Much incontinence can be cured, some improved, or, at the worst, much better managed. The continence adviser will assess patients when requested, or act in an advisory capacity to other professionals, individuals or organisations. The adviser needs to work closely with other members of the primary health care team, as a multi-disciplinary approach is often needed to solve the problem. The role of the continence adviser is threefold.

1.   *A source of reference*, as the adviser has a wide knowledge of what aids are available on the market, what methods of management may be used, what new drugs are available, where special incontinence clinics are situated and what current research is revealing.

2.   *To promote continence*. This is achieved by disseminating the relevant information to those who suffer, those who care for them in whatever capacity, and to the general public. The message is that help is available and must be sought and demanded, also that prevention is better than a cure.

3.   *To endeavour to change attitudes about incontinence*. NO ONE should be told that they must put up with the situation, because, with careful assessment, the use of drugs, toileting regimes and pelvic floor exercises many can achieve continence.

Where there is no continence adviser, the district nurse or health visitor should be able to help. Some general practitioners are very good with advice about incontinence problems. Education for all is the key word.

Practical aspects of promoting continence

Home and clothing adaptations. Sometimes incontinence is caused because the individual receives insufficient warning to allow him to reach and use the toilet in time. This may be due to many factors – for example, poor mobility, nerve impairment, an ageing or unstable bladder. There may also be problems in removing and replacing clothing during the toileting procedure. This should always be carefully observed, any difficulties being obvious in a functional assessment of daily living. In these cases home adaptations and adapted clothing may help to improve matters. Occupational therapists should be actively involved in these areas. In some places, equipment and clothing may be tried at a local aids centre.

Personal hygiene and odour control. Freshly passed urine is not offensive unless there is a problem, as odour only begins when the urine starts to decompose on contact with the air. Soiled and wet clothing and linen need rinsing in cold water as soon as possible, and if it is not practical to wash them immediately they should be immersed in a bucket of cold water. Wet pads should be changed frequently to minimise skin and odour problems.

Ideally skin should be washed at each pad change, but a minimum of washing night and morning should be encouraged. Not everyone is able to use the bath, or afford the hot water for daily baths, but there are several portable bidets on the market which fit into the top of the toilet and may be a practical alternative. Perfumed talcum powder and soap and bath additives should be avoided, as these may cause skin irritation. If soreness does occur a good barrier cream should be applied. This should be available on prescription. Where there is a problem with odour in clothes, carpets or rooms, a good deodoriser can be used either directly upon problem areas or in the water used for laundry and washing floors. It may also be used directly on the pad. One drop is usually sufficient. These products are available from chemists. Fungicidal powders may also help to mask odour if sprinkled on to a pad.

Menstrual care. This is an added problem for women. Tampons are a very good method to use, providing that she is not handicapped and unable to use them, as they do not interfere with the pads used for incontinence. However, if this method is not possible the incontinence pads should be changed much more frequently. In either case scrupulous attention to personal hygiene is essential. Vaginal deodorants are not to be recommended as they can cause skin irritation.

Disposal of pads. Under no circumstances should these pads be flushed down the toilet. Most of them are not intended for this method of disposal and neither is our sewage system designed to cope with them. Neither should most pads be burned at home, as they are highly inflammable and the waterproof backing may give off noxious fumes. Some areas have special medical waste collection services separate from the normal domestic refuse collection; others burn all refuse anyway, but if the local authority has neither of these services, ask them for advice on disposal, or wrap each pad well in newspaper and seal several of them in a polythene bag before placing in the dustbin.

Laundry services. Some areas provide this service for incontinent people, and each area will vary in what it supplies. The service is usually run by the social service department, health authority, or as a joint venture. There are normally set criteria as to who should receive help. Provision is variable and it is best to enquire at the local clinic or town hall.

What may be done to help?

Most of the following are common sense and do not need special training. However, other disciplines need to be consulted over management.

1.   *Medical examination*. The client should see his own doctor to exclude medical causes.

2.   *Fluid intake* should be checked as many incontinent people cut down on their intake in the mistaken belief that they will need to 'go' less often. This merely encourages a small capacity bladder and may make the problem worse. If there is nothing medically wrong a fluid intake of three to five pints daily is recommended. Sometimes it has been found that the drinking of vast quantities may cause incontinence especially if mobility is restricted. Tea, coffee and cocoa all contain caffeine which acts as a mild diuretic, thus a de-caffeinated drink may need to be substituted or a bland alternative.

3.   *The diet* should be checked. An inadequate diet may cause constipation, and this together with lack of exercise and poor mobility can cause incontinence as a full rectum presses on the bladder and diminishes the capacity and sensation. A diet containing fresh fruit and vegetables and more fibre should be encouraged; but beware – a high fibre diet needs plenty of liquid! Where there are problems of constipation the general practitioner should be approached.

4.   *Exercise* should be encouraged, particularly for elderly people who tend to sit for long periods. Mobility around the home should be encouraged and where there are problems the community physiotherapist will be able to advise, if one is available in the area (see Chapter 8).

5.   *Pelvic floor exercises* often help, even in severe cases. These sound impressive, but are *simple* and can be done by both men and women.[4] The aim is to tighten up the deep muscles of the pelvic floor which may have become lax through

childbirth or persistently straining at stool. It must be stressed that it can be two or three months before results are seen. The local physiotherapy department may run classes for these exercises, or the community physiotherapist may visit and advise the client.

6.   *Record episodes* of wetness, times of emptying the bladder and the amount passed. This may indicate where the problem lies, i.e. use of diuretics, overnight sedation, sitting too long or definite bladder malfunction. The chart may indicate if toileting regimes or bladder re-training need to be given.

Aids available

There are a wide variety of aids available to help manage incontinence. These include commodes, urinals (male and female), bed pans and chemical toilets. These should be available either through the health authority, social service departments or the Red Cross home nursing service. Community nursing services may provide some bedding protection as well as pads and pants, and advise on condom drainage.

Male aids. The choice of any form of management depends upon individual preference if it is to be used successfully. A male urinal may be all that is necessary. These are of polypropelene and are easily cleaned and sterilised and are available from retail chemists. There are a number of collecting devices which are worn attached to the penis, and the urine is collected into a legworn drainage bag which can be emptied by means of a tap at the bottom (care must be taken that this is closed before use). The continence adviser, district nurse or local surgical fitter will measure and fit these appliances as careful fitting is essential to avoid leakage. Leg bags last five to seven days and should be rinsed thoroughly daily. A hypochlorite solution may be used for this. Sheaths are usually changed daily but may last longer. Great care must be given to the skin. All of these are available on prescription from the general practitioner.

For the man who 'dribbles' a little there are several 'drip' collectors on the market, which are available by mail order and not on prescription. Boots also retail a male pouch which is useful for 'dribblers', either used alone or with a small pad.

Female aids. There are several urinals available which are shaped to accommodate the female anatomy, but all need care and practice to use successfully. They may be available through the health authority, otherwise from mail order firms. Apart from catheters, pads and pants there are no other female aids available.

Pads and pants. All health authorities provide some incontinence materials, but may limit the supply to those in receipt of nursing care only, or the supply may be very limited and not suitable for all types of incontinence.

Pants are of three types as follows:

1.   Marsupial. These have an outside pouch which is water-proof and which will hold a disposable pad.
2.   Stretch mesh. These are semi-disposable and will hold a waterproof backed pad in place.
3.   Waterproof. These are usually plastic or latex.

All pants must fit snugly to the body, otherwise the pads do not absorb urine efficiently. Some pants are made to look like 'Y' fronts which give a more acceptable image for men and they do not look like knickers on the washing line.

A pouch type of pant is also made with a drop front or as side-opening models which may be of help to those who are handicapped, or those caring for an incontinent person.

No pants should be bleached or boiled in the wash, as this destroys the waterproofing and stretch materials.

Pads fall into four categories:

1.   Those for light incontinence.
2.   Those for medium incontinence – both of these may have waterproof backs and may also be used for faecal soiling.
3.   Those for heavy or double incontinence all of which are water-proof backed.
4.   An all-in-one garment of either a pull on or diaper type with protective backings.

Many pads are made with the layer next to the skin acting as a one-way fabric which should keep the individual dry. If it does not, either the pad is inadequate for the amount of urine being produced, it is not being changed often enough, or the pants do not fit closely enough to hold the pad in the correct position. Many chemists are now starting to stock incontinence material. Boots, for instance, have a large range available under their own label. However, these pads and pants are usually expensive. The Disabled Living Foundation can supply details together with a list of resource centres. Details of most available aids for managing incontinence can be found in handbooks produced by The Association of Continence Advisers.[5]

Stoma care

The most common conditions requiring a stoma are as follows:

The older age group:	Diverticular disease; malignant tumours of the large bowel; malignance of the urinary bladder.
Teenagers and young adults:	Ulcerative colitis; Crohn's disease; Inflammatory conditions of the bowel.
Babies and children:	Congenital abnormalities; spina bifida; imperforated anus; Hirschsprungs disease; urinary bladder abnormalities; kidney abnormalities.

Other causes include trauma, multiple sclerosis; the latter sometimes causing double incontinence. In some areas nurses specialising in stoma care are appointed. Their main aim is to rehabilitate the patient to as high a degree of self-sufficiency as possible, and to build an informal, friendly relationship with patients and relatives. Not only are the physical requirements considered but also the psychological and social trauma associated with the dysfunction and disfigurement which accompanies a stoma. An assessment of individual physical and psychological needs is made and a holistic approach to care provided to meet these needs. Patients need to be counselled before and after surgery with reassurance and encouragement being given so that they are able to resume their normal way of life as soon as possible. When this special type of surgery is explained, many patients find it inconceivable that they will spend the remainder of their lives with an adhesive plastic bag stuck to their abdomen, containing urine or faeces, although in a few cases this may be a temporary measure so that certain healing processes can take place. However, it is often much less traumatic for a patient or his carer to empty or change the bag, than to have the discomfort or embarrassment of incontinence, or frequently being lifted from chair to lavatory. In the majority of cases this gives the patient more independence, especially when going out and about. The patient with a stoma must be reassured that, with a properly fitting appliance, there will be no smell, apart from when the bag is changed. The occupational therapist can help in reassuring patients of this and alerting the nurse if problems do arise.

Other fears that the patients may have are: will they be disabled; can they resume their employment; will a special diet be necessary; can they have a bath?; can they swim or engage in sporting activities?; will their sexual life be affected?; will social life be non-existent? All these questions and many more can be discussed in confidence and positive assurance given.

Appliances

The range of available stoma appliances are numerous. There are still a number of people who use the older type of rubber bags; however, these must be kept scrupulously clean to avoid odour. Most people now prefer to use the plastic disposable type. Although it must always be remembered that the type the patient wishes to use is the most important one to him.

The disposable appliance must *not* be flushed down the toilet or burned on a domestic fire. In most areas there is a special collection service, or if that is not the person's wishes, they may be taught a simple method of emptying the bag and disposing of this in the domestic disposal service – dustbin. According to the Department of Environmental Health, this is quite acceptable.

All appliances and accessories are available on prescription. Patients with a permanent stoma and who normally pay prescription charges are able to obtain an exemption certificate from the local general practitioners committee.

Support groups

These are just starting to spring up around the country. The local reference library, social service department or community nursing service will be able to give details of any local groups.

Common sense is the best attribute for dealing with incontinence allied to a sound assessment backed by a knowledge of normal physiology and available resources. Together they should produce a much improved quality of life for any sufferer.

Acknowledgements. My thanks go to my colleague, Mrs Pat Rennie, Stoma Care Sister, for her help with the section on Stoma Care.

References

1. Thomas, Plymat, Meade, Blannin, 'The prevalence of urinary incontinence', *British Medical Journal,* Vol. 281, 8 November 1980.
2. Thomas, Egan, Walgrove, Meade, 'The prevalence of faecal and double incontinence', *Community Medicine* Vol. 6, pp. 216–220, 1984.
3. *The Problem of Promoting Continence,* report published by Squibb Surgicare in conjunction with The Royal College of Nursing, 1983.
4. D. Mandlestam, *Incontinence and its management,* Heinemann.
5. The Association of Continence Advisers, *Directory of Aids* (2nd edition), Disabled Living Foundation, 380–384 Harrow Road, London W9 2HU.

Further Reading

B. Breckman, Ed., *Stoma Care.* Beaconsfield Publishers, 1981.

R. C. L. Feneley and J. P. Blannin, *Incontinence, A Patient Handbook.* Churchill Livingstone, 1984.

M. Swash. 'New concepts in incontinence', *British Medical Journal,* Vol. 290, 5 January 1985.

Action on Incontinence, King's Fund Publications, 1983.

Stoma Therapy Review, Coroplast Ltd, Bridge House, Orchard Lane, Huntingdon, Cambridge, PE18 6QT.

Chapter 14

Maintaining mental health

LESLEY FORD
Community Occupational Therapist, Maidstone

The maintenance of mental health in the community is probably the newest and intrinsically dynamic field of occupational therapy practise in the 1980s. The enormous social and therapeutic demands for care in the community can be traced back to the 1950s. Development of new drug treatments, two Mental Health Acts (1959 and 1983) and subsequent documents and White Papers[1] are directing the prevention, treatment and rehabilitation services for the mentally ill away from institutional care, to the community.

The traditional medical model of treatment is no longer considered to be the most appropriate for all psychiatric referrals, and the collaborative skills of multidisciplinary teamwork are more geared to meet many current circumstances and needs.[2]

For occupational therapists working in the community, the most significant parts of the Mental Act 1983 are those relating to guardianship and to aftercare. The Act reinforces the statutory duty of both health and social services to provide aftercare for those patients who have been detained under Sections 3 and 37, and to provide preventative care and treatment in the community for those under guardianship.

Early research and information programmes

Although other professions have been treating the mentally ill in the community for some years, it is only now that the role of occupational therapy in this field is being recognised and fully developed.

Research and development programmes are limited but some early work is currently being undertaken and should be mentioned.

1. Investigation into the role of the occupational therapist in group homes and hostels.[3]

2. A realistic appraisal of the functioning of a day clinic to enable future planning and services to develop effectively in response to changing local needs and attitudes.[4]

3. Early reports of the beginning of community-based occupational therapy services.[5]

4. A Cambridge-based research therapist is planning programmes in the following areas:

    (a) A survey of admission ward user's views about their mental health needs and observations in the context of their admission, support systems and preference for source of help. This investigation aims to establish some hypotheses about the needs for community services.

    (b) Future pilot project to evaluate the effectiveness of a relaxation/anxiety management group as an alternative to first time prescribing of minor tranquillisers by the GP.

    (c) Follow-up of work done by the home management unit.

Membership of multiprofessional groups working in this sphere gives the therapist a broader view of overall non-statutory planning and practises on a national scale. Valuable support and information can also be gained and exchanged through the agencies listed at the end of this chapter.

Work situations

Community Services have been criticised for developing without a common philosophy,[6] and of being piece-meal and non complementary.[7] Colleagues in this speciality may be employed by the NHS, by local authorities or be in a joint funded post according to local planning and resources. In all situations the occupational therapist can only practise successfully as a fully integrated member of a multidisciplinary team. Variations of setting may be any of the following:

1. *Hospital-based community teams.*

    (a) Acute mental illness team.

    (b) Continuing care team.

        (c) Elderly mentally ill team.
2.   *Satellite day resources.*
        (a) Day hospital.
        (b) Day unit.
        (c) Day centre.
        (d) Sheltered workshop.

In these posts the therapist has a permanent base at the unit and carries out much of the group and individual treatment programmes there. Home visits are made where appropriate.

3.   *Community mental health teams*

These are office-based teams in a range of locations which function more broadly in the open community. The travelling day hospital could be one concept. Teams use a variety of local resources, e.g. patients' home, church halls, clinic, group homes, voluntary agencies accommodation, etc. or wherever is most appropriate.

4.   *Community care team*

The member of this team is a generic occupational therapist working from a GP health centre base.

Needs, resources, skills

The common need of all clients is to maintain optimum mental health, and effective functioning in life skills to sustain their role in society.

The potential demand upon community services can be overwhelming to an occupational therapist setting up a new post, and the following guidelines may be helpful.

1.   *Initial action*
        (a) study local policies and planning;
        (b) discuss apparent areas of need with medical staff, social workers, community nurses and other occupational therapist colleagues;
        (c) survey established resources;
        (d) invite and assess referrals.
2.   *Subsequent action*
        (a) define own skills and role in relation to referrals;
        (b) survey potential resources;
        (c) initiate treatment programmes and develop appropriate group therapies;
        (d) identify support system for self.

It has been said that a good occupational therapist working in community mental health should be 'up front, laid back and altogether'. This very concise description could be expanded to describe the following:

1. *Personal qualities*
    (a) Maturity (not related to age).
    (b) Self motivated and self reliant.
    (c) Innovative and communicative.
    (e) Non judgemental, flexible and empathetic.
2. *Skills required*
    (a) Knowledge and experience in medical field.
    (b) Counselling.
    (c) Group skills.
    (d) Management skills.
    (e) Social skills.
    (f) Public speaking and public relations abilities.
3. *Post registration training* in:
    (a) Further counselling.
    (b) Family therapy.
    (c) Research techniques.
    (d) Appropriate law, and political and local government policies.
    (e) Specific skills as appropriate.

Treatment media

The treatment media used in this specialised area of work will be relatively consistent throughout the wide range of situations. Variations will occur according to the individual skills of the therapist, the skills and involvement of other members of the team, and the current needs of the mentally ill people in the catchment area. Availability of suitable resources and staffing levels are also relevant factors.

Table 4 was compiled after the first meeting of the Special Interest Group of Occupational Therapists in 1981, which was attended by twenty-two occupational therapists working outside the hospital setting. It is too early to record an updated comparison, but after ten years perhaps another table would indicate whether there have been any significant changes in the therapeutic role.

Whether the focus of therapy is prophylactic or rehabilitative,

Table 4 The numbers and percentage of community occupational therapists who use specific treatment activities.

Activity	Yes		No	
	Numbers	%	Numbers	%
Home management	19	86	3	14
Social skills training	19	86	3	14
Relaxation training	17	77	5	23
Physical fitness	14	64	8	36
Creative therapy (projective techniques)	13	59	9	41
Family work	15	68	7	32
Counselling	16	73	6	27
Self-help groups	12	55	10	45
Encouraging use of normal social activities	21	95	1	5
Crisis intervention	13	59	9	41
Occupational therapy assessments	21	95	1	5
Advising other disciplines/agencies	16	73	6	27
Group homes, hostels	13	59	9	41
Day centres	18	82	4	18

each person's treatment programme should be individually planned in consultation with him/her. Some time scale, or anticipated number of sessions should be mentioned in the early stages. A realisation and commitment by the client to the aims of the therapeutic programme will prevent occupational therapy visits from being perceived as social 'coffee and chat' sessions.

The treatment media used have been divided into five main sections:

1.   Individual treatments

Occupational therapy assessment. This should be a holistic assessment of the person's mental health and lifestyle, and the treatment and support needed to enable him to function at maximum level.

Home management assessment/training programmes. This sphere of therapeutic need may be found across the whole range of probable referrals, ages and illness patterns. 'Non-judgemental' should be the keyword for every therapist preparing for a home assessment visit. The therapist must be extremely sensitive to the family dynamics throughout the involvement. Of course, there are unacceptable standards of habitation but there should be a clear distinction between occupational therapist intervention to introduce more effective domestic routines, and disturbing a whole family's way of life. Some situations do indicate the need for a therapeutic family commitment to help and support the vulnerable member. On the other hand the family may need re-educating to tactfully withdraw gradually and allow the member greater independence and responsibility. Examples like this may occur when a husband recently retired or made redundant unconsciously takes over the home management role. This can lead to confusion and anxiety for the partner, sometimes precipitating an acute illness.

Relaxation. Individual sessions may be indicated if a person is too anxious initially to join group sessions. Other indications for individual therapy may occur owing to geographical and social difficulties.

Socialisation. The therapist should be very clear about her own philosophies of community care. In this circumstance the therapist should act as a guide and facilitator rather than a leader and initiator. An extensive knowledge of all available community resources will enable her to encourage her clients to develop the skills and confidence to use them fully. Too much emphasis on sheltered day care and social groups could lead to the development of an institutionalised framework in the community. The building of successful relationships should develop confidence among vulnerable people and encourage them together to develop their social lives more fully.

Assessment of the elderly. This is usually part of a multidisciplinary assessment, taking a holistic view of the physical, psychiatric and social needs of the person. In many areas specialist psychogeriatric teams are being developed to meet the specific needs of this expanding client group. It has long been recognised that to remove the elderly person from his familiar environment precipitates confusion and disorientation, so care in the home environment is clearly indicated whenever possible.

Counselling. This is an integral component of every therapeutic relationship. However, the community occupational therapist has a further need to extend her knowledge of the principle, dynamics and practice of counselling to enhance her effectiveness to meet the specific needs. The most common situations requiring empathic counselling skills are most likely to be marital/relationship problems, sexual problems and cases of bereavement and loss.

Behavioural therapies. Treatment programmes should be individually tailored to the behaviour patterns which are presented by the patient. The occupational therapist is most likely to be involved in phobic desensitisation, assertiveness training and anxiety management.

2.   Group treatments

Group therapies have been described as being '. . . where sociological or psychological concepts are being used to motivate local people to learn how to work together to bring about some change in their situation.'[8] They have been differentiated as being task orientated with specific goals, a process orientated and directed to group fulfilment. Community occupational therapists involved in group therapy will often be co-working with a member of another profession.

These programmes include the following:

Social skills; personal effectiveness; assertiveness. The formation of all these groups depends upon current needs which do vary considerably without any specific pattern. Careful assessment of members for a closed group, planning a suitably orientated programme and sufficient preparation for each session are all necessary requirements. Real settings, role play and the use of video may all enhance the value of the community situation.

Relaxation; anxiety management. Both of these groups are similar in their aims and method. Yoga sessions or group relaxation sessions are widely used as an important therapeutic medium. At one end of the scale they may be perceived as socio-therapeutic activities; whereas at the other the psychotherapuetic techniques of anxiety management teach the necessary responses to counteract anxiety and gradually expose the client to the imagined threat, proving that he can cope.

A new concept is to develop an anxiety management programme as an alternative treatment to the first time prescription of tranquillisers. Experimental groups are recording their work. (See Appendix I, Anxiety Management.)

Phobic groups. Specifically orientated groups working towards individual goals for each member.

Creative therapies, projective techniques. These therapies, more usually associated with hospital occupational therapy, are sometimes developed for group work in community situations.

Other groups are developed to meet local needs and where the appropriately skilled therapists are available.

These might include:

Loss group. This may be needed to meet the requirements of a small number of people who are suffering loss from bereavement or redundancy. The group aims to enable people to express their feelings, to understand them, to work through them and eventually to re-establish their life in its new situation.

Womens group. A group to explore issues particular to women. An open forum to express feelings and exchange views and experiences with other women. These groups are usually lively and often creative in outcome.

Mothers group. Several experimental groups set up across the country have proved very beneficial to the members. The purpose is to enable mothers experiencing neuroses to explore their problems, examine their relationships and attitudes, and seek some changes. As many mothers referred to these groups have babies or pre-school age children, special provision needs to be made for their care during group discussion time. Allowance should also be made for some social time to observe the interaction between mothers and their children. This could offer valuable insight. Closed group discussion encourages the development of a safe confidential environment allowing these anxious and often isolated mothers the opportunity to explore all the facets of their current problems. Mutual support enables them to seek suitable changes to improve their situations.

3.   Involvement with other agencies

The occupational therapist working in the community is often in contact with other agencies. In certain circumstances the therapist may be even more closely involved, attending meetings, assisting with groups, introducing new members or even be an organiser. In this context the agencies could be:

MIND

National Schizophrenia Fellowship

Anorexic Family Aid

Libra

Alcoholics Anonymous

Age Concern

The Association of Post-Natal Illness

Drug dependency groups

In another sphere of work the therapist will be working with the many agencies involved with housing. Local authority housing, Part III accommodation, housing associations, hostels, and housing co-operatives are all alternatives to private housing. Although finding new accommodation for a client is traditionally seen as being within the role of the social worker the occupational therapist is becoming more involved in assessing and preparing people to cope with a new lifestyle. People leaving hospital after many years as an in-patient need very thorough preparation and support if they are to adapt successfully to independent living.

4.   Non-structured groups

A community care programme should allow for periods of non-structured support as a very important component. Whilst not being directly therapeutic they play an invaluable role in maintaining mental health. For example, one mental health centre has nominated three days per week for structured therapeutic sessions and two days are reserved as support days.

Everyday life is not totally structured, neither do all referrals to the service require specific therapeutic input. Generalised day care offers support, and drop-in facilities and open sessions are other models. Support sessions offer the client the opportunity to maintain low-key contact with staff; to make and maintain relationships; a respite from sometimes tense home situations; and to seek help and advice when necessary. For the staff there is an opportunity to observe the person's general welfare and pick up any significant signals.

With some initial professional guidance, sessions can develop into valuable self help groups which could be meaningful and productive. Client-arranged outings, money raising events, and charity work are all potential activities, as are the sharing of skills in leisure, sport and recreation.

In this section some mention should also be made of relatives support groups and their contribution to the welfare of the carers. Groups for the carers of the elderly mentally ill, and of schizophrenic people offer an opportunity for the relations to receive support for themselves.

5. Work orientation

With the high levels of unemployment current today, the therapeutic power of work-orientated groups cannot be over estimated. As a final goal in rehabilitation they can offer a closely realistic lifestyle for many people, whilst retaining a sheltered aspect. For the successful person, suitable work groups could provide the final stage in total rehabilitation to open employment.

A great variety of groups are operating successfully in the community, offering work routines, status, and increasing self esteem to disadvantaged people.

Readers may wish to acquire further knowledge of co-operatives; horticultural groups (some functioning as co-operatives); industrial therapy; clerical assessment and rehabilitation groups; sheltered workshops; community work groups; voluntary skills groups.

The occupational therapist working to maintain mental health in the community will have the potential to develop a role according to personal initiatives and local needs. Using a wide range of therapeutic media, and working in a variety of locations, the therapist should offer an effective preventative treatment and rehabilitation occupational therapy service to the mentally ill.

Acknowledgements. My thanks go to my colleagues Catherine Wells and Lesley Wright for their help with this chapter and in particular for their contribution to the appendices which follow.

Appendix I – Anxiety management

Anxiety is a complex condition, one that creates a confusing and frightening experience for the sufferer which affects their entire life. It produces distressing physical symptoms, adversely affects personal relationships and behaviour in public; and also severely limits the sufferer's freedom. People can be helped either on their own or within a group, by helping them to understand the physiology of the condition and recognise the symptoms produced.

Physiology of anxiety

On occasions such as speaking formally in public or prior to taking an important examination, most people recall physical sensations such as a pounding of the heart, or 'butterflies' in the stomach. Here the mind registers danger, causing the nervous system to send out impulses which energise the body in an attempt to cope with the situation. In an anxiety state, however, the nervous system is triggered in response to no obvious source of external danger. It is reassuring for those people experiencing anxiety states to learn that distressing bodily reactions are normal and not harmful, but are happening in abnormal circumstances.

Recognition of the symptoms of anxiety

To assist in the recognition of symptoms and promoting an understanding of the situations that trigger off reactions, the introduction of a diary recording behaviour and physical problems can be helpful. This involves noting carefully problems that are experienced along with the intensity of reaction on a scale of 1–5.

Teaching responses to counteract anxiety

An important part of the process of recovering from anxiety entails teaching the bodily responses which counteract it. To facilitate this, it is helpful for the therapist to present a variety of relaxation techniques as individuals will differ in approaches they find effective. Details of relaxation techniques are listed in the References.

Exposure to anxiety provoking situations

The motto for facing threatening situations is 'Challenge but not overwhelm'. A situation from the diary can indicate what gave rise to mild anxiety. This can be set as an initial target and practised daily with the aid of relaxation techniques. Once comfortable and confident with that situation, progression can be gradually made to more demanding ones.

Appendix II – Anorexia

Anorexic Family Aid (AFA) is a self help support group for sufferers of anorexia and bulimia nervosa and their families. It was established in 1976, in Norwich, and registered as a charity, with a board of trustees to oversee the management of the group.

Anorexic Family Aid provides regular meetings for those suffering from, or interested in, eating disorders. The objects of the group meetings are to educate and involve those attending, thus encouraging families and individuals to look at their own situations, and to understand the disorders and to find their own ways of coping with them. The regularity of the meetings is important, so that sufferers know that support is available both from the team working at AFA, and from other involved families. There is an extensive library at the group, which is well used and provides books, tapes of talks and a video made by AFA.

The office is able to provide support to members both through the telephone and by mail. All letters are individually responded to, and support may continue in this way if the member lives far away. A monthly newsletter is circulated to ensure that isolated members are kept in touch, and the staff are available through the week to talk on the telephone.

Anorexic Family Aid exists not only to help those people currently suffering from anorexia and bulimia, but also to educate others about the disorders, as early recognition and prompt help can influence the length of time the illness takes. In 1984 following many enquiries from outside the region, the need to establish a national information centre was recognised. The DHSS provided a three-year grant for AFA to set up and run an information centre based in Norwich, which aims to collect and collate information from sufferers and professionals throughout the country. Membership to the centre includes quarterly newsletters, telephone and letter support, and advice about facilities in the area.

The aim of Anorexic Family Aid is not to provide treatment; it provides a forum for a greater understanding of anorexia and bulimia nervosa to take place, and it enables sufferers to gain support and help from each other as well as from the skilled team working within the organisation.

Appendix III – Setting up a group

Identify the group. It is necessary to highlight areas of need. These are established by assessing presenting problems from the clients referred, and liaising with colleagues. Those with common areas of need can be effectively grouped together. For example, women with reactive depression and anxiety, between the ages of 30 and 50 years; or young people with poor social skills.

Define the aims of the group, including the direction which the group should progress and its anticipated outcome. At this stage the aims need not be expressed in precise behavioural terminology, but rather used to give a generalised direction for the group.

For example, the aims for a relaxation group may be:

(a)   to encourage members to gain insights into their stress situations, and the underlying conflicts contributing towards their state of anxiety;

(b)   to gain an understanding of their responses to fear;

(c)   to gain relief from the symptoms of anxiety;

(d)   to develop an attitude of mutual support and self help.

Determine the staffing of the group. The necessity for the presence of a co-therapist will need to be considered, as will the need for the involvement of volunteers especially if creche facilities are needed.

Determine the size of the group. Bearing in mind the specific needs of the group, and the established aims, the number of participants can be set. For example:

i   A group aimed at encouraging mutual self disclosure and facilitate emotional expression may only cater for up to eight members

ii   A group aiming to encourage communication skills through remedial drama may cater for around twelve.

Decide on the time period for which the group should run. Specific skills may only need a short period of six or eight sessions whereas others, such as self-help groups, may last for any length of time. Alternatively, a number of sessions may need to be followed by a review with assessment of progress and determining future aims.

Decide whether the group should be open or closed. Where the development of trusting and supportive relationships with other group members are of prime importance, a closed group may be appropriate. An open group allows opportunities for new referrals benefiting from such an experience, and joining an already established group.

Structure the timing of group sessions. It can be helpful to form guidelines as to how sessions will be structured. For example, a two-hourly anxiety management group could be structured as follows:
> *Welcome.* Informal chat whilst group members arrive (10 minutes).
> *Teaching.* The physiology of anxiety/techniques for coping (40 minutes).
> *Coffee break.*
> *Discussion.* Opportunity for mutual sharing and support (60 minutes).

Organise the venue. An appropriate location will need to be sought and booked, ensuring that it offers the necessary facilities.

Request referrals (if needed). A letter stating briefly the aims and nature of the group can be circulated to the relevant referring agencies.

Individually assess all clients referred. To determine appropriateness for the group. If the referral is considered inappropriate then suggestions should be offered for alternative treatment. It is important that the referring agency is informed of the outcome of the assessment.

Establish the group. At this point commitment to the group must be discussed with each referred person. This will include such matters as attending for the full duration of the group, and taking responsibility for bringing important personal issues to it.

References

1. DHSS, *Better Services for the Mentally Ill*. London: Department of Health and Social Service, 1975.
2. Helena Waters and John Sturt, 'Role of the psychiatrist in community based mental health care. *The Lancet*, 12 March 1985.
3. E. J. Downing. *Report on the Role of OT in Group Homes* and *Report Looking at Role of OT within a DHSS Resettlement Hostel*, Lambeth Social Services, 1981.
4. Gill Westland, *A Study of the Work of the Cambridge Day Clinic*, British *Journal of Occupational Therapy*, Vol. 45, No. 9, pp. 304–5.
5. M. Crawford, *Occupational Therapy for the Mentally Ill at Home*, Hammersmith and Fulham Social Services, 1981.
   L. Ford, *Evalulation of the Need for a Community Occupational Therapy Service in Psychiatry*, Norwich Health District, 1982.
6. Social Services Committee Enquiry, *Community Care with Special Reference to Adult Mentally Ill and Mentally Handicapped*, 1984.
7. C. A. Butterworth and D. Skidmore, *Caring for Mentally Ill in the Community*, Croom Helm Ltd, 1981.
8. S. Thompson and J. H. Kahn, *The Group Process as a Helping Technique*. Introduction by Dame Eileen Younghusband. Pergamman Press, 1970.

Further reading

College of Occupational Therapists, *Community Care, with Special Reference to Adult Mentally Ill and Mentally Handicapped People, Social Services Committee Inquiry*, 1984.
D. Goldberg and P. Huxley, *Mental Illness in the Community: the pathways to psychiatric care*, London: Tavistock Publications, 1980.
The Rising Tide: Developing Services for Mental Illness in Old Age, Health Advisory Service, 1982.
Nancy Wansborough and Philip Cooper, *Open Employment after Mental Illness*, London: Tavistock Publications, 1980.
M. Wilson, *Occupational Therapy in Short Term Psychiatry*, Churchill-Livingstone, 1984.
J. K. Wing and B. Morris, *Handbook of Psychiatric Rehabilitation*, London: Oxford University Press, 1981.

Useful addresses

Interdisciplinary Association of Mental Health Workers, 126 Albert Street, London NW1.

Good Practices in Mental Health Project, 67 Kentish Town Road, London NW1 8NY.

MIND, 22 Harley Street, London W1N 2ED.

Creative Day Care, Studdert Kennedy Centre, Worcester.

Relaxation for Living, 29 Burwood Park Road, Walton-on-Thames, Surrey KT12 5LH. (093-22 27826). Provides information cassette tapes, and runs groups in many parts of the country.

Stress Syndrome Foundation, Cedar House, Yalding, Kent, ME18 6JD (0622 814431). Supplies information on stress-related problems.

Phobics Society, 4 Cheltenham Road, Manchester M21 1Q2. (061-881 1937). Advises on any type of phobia.

Open Door Association, 447 Pensby Road, Heswall, Wirral L61 9PQ (051-648 2022). Helps sufferers of agoraphobia.

Lifestyle Training Centre, 23 Abingdon Road, London W8 (01-938 1011). Supplies books and cassette tapes on relaxation and coping with anxiety, depression and phobias.

Wheel of Yoga, 80 Leckhampton Road, Cheltenham, Gloucestershire, GL53 0BN.

Health Education Council, 78 New Oxford Street, London WC1 1AH (01-637 1881).

Chapter 15

Occupational therapy and mental handicap

CHIA SWEE HONG
Occupational Therapist, Norwich

DAWN PATTERSON
Occupational Therapist, Lambeth Community Assessment and Treatment Team, London

It is now generally accepted that all people with a mental handicap are capable of some learning. It is also accepted that for the majority it is appropriate for them to be cared for at home rather than in an institution. Consequently community facilities for mentally handicapped people are gradually improving, albeit slowly. The provision of services in many areas, though, is still based on the philosophy and interest of the people providing them with hospitals continuing to house the majority of mentally handicapped people supposedly needing care and support. Those people who are in the community tend to be less severely handicapped and live in purpose-built hostels and group homes. Other means of providing care include fostering services and lodgings. Community villages such as L'Arche and CARE (Cottage and Rural Enterprises Ltd.) also offer positive caring and living environments committed to serving the needs of the individual.[1,2]

Developments that have come about are influenced by a number of factors such as the White Paper *Better Services for the Mentally Handicapped*;[3] the work of the National Development Group and the Development Team for the Mentally Handicapped; changes in professional attitudes; and demands made by those individuals and organisations concerned with mentally handicapped people.

Another strong impact is 'the principle of normalisation'[4] from Scandinavia which advocates the rights and provisions of services and facilities for mentally handicapped people to live as normally as possible, i.e. in a family environment, which might also include work and social opportunities. However, without adequate supporting services the mentally handicapped person may become overwhelmed with the competition that he may have to face especially when competing for accommodation and work.

Better Services for the Mentally Handicapped emphasised the need for local community-based services and the development teams for the mentally handicapped which were subsequently established in 1976 introduced the concepts of the community mental handicap team (CMHT) and the community mental handicap unit (CMHU) as essential elements in the establishment of a local service for people with a mental handicap.

The community mental handicap teams

During the past ten years the development of CMHTs has been well documented on a national level with many models of practice described. However, different districts have established teams according to their resources and the specific needs of the clients in their charge which has led to diversification from the original recommended model.[5] The development team recommended that one CMHT should serve a population of between 60,000 and 80,000.

A CMHT usually consists of 'core' members who include a consultant psychiatrist, nurse and social worker. Speech therapy, physiotherapy, occupational therapy and psychology are all included to a greater or lesser extent. The team carries out most of their work in the client's home and working place with therapeutic sessions taking place in an appropriate situation.

The aims of the team are as follows:

1.   To provide a service for mentally handicapped adults through a multi-disciplinary assessment and treatment programme based within the community which is both comprehensive and responsive to the individual's needs.

2.   To offer guidance and advice to individuals, families and groups concerned with the mentally handicapped.

3.   To encourage and maintain independence within the com-

munity by offering regular assistance, guidance and special-ist skills.

4.   To provide training and education to parents, carers, mem-bers of other professions and volunteers.

5.   To provide support and advice to other services, thus enabling the mentally handicapped to make the fullest use of them.

6.   To contribute to the planning of services for the mentally handicapped.

The team's philosophy is based on 'normalisation', therefore the referral system might well be informal, encouraging the mentally handicapped people to refer themselves. Once identified as mentally handicapped, they remain the concern of the local services for the duration of their lives or until such a time that they move from the district.

The team meets regularly to discuss new referrals and to allocate key workers who can act as the link with each family; and to discuss policy matters and any relevant issues. Clearly, communication within the team is of major importance if this approach is to be effective in practice. Joint visits are sometimes necessary as this facilitates an intimate understanding of each profession's skills and the contribution that each can offer thus forming a valuable founda-tion for team work.

The role of occupational therapy

In contrast to existing information on CMHTs, there is very little documentation on the role of occupational therapy. This role incorporates a wide range of skills including both physical and psychological functioning. This is specifically highlighted when working with those who have additional disabilities to their mental handicap such as psychiatric disorders, sensory deficits, behavioural or emotional problems or physical handicaps.

Thus the role of the occupational therapist is to:

(a)   assess sensory and motor skills; play, self help, perceptual, social, work and leisure skills;

(b)   devise therapy programmes to meet the needs of the client which could include both individual and group work;

(c)   assess and provide aids and equipment and to teach the client and his carers in their use;

(d)   provide a counselling service to those concerned in his care;
(e)   offer advice concerning the home and surrounding environment including mobility;
(f)   provide support to carers through seminars and support groups and liaise with sources of expertise/information where appropriate;
(g)   encourage parents, relatives and others to participate fully with the programme;
(h)   help educate the community with regards to the needs of handicapped people

Clinical work may be divided into two categories, direct and indirect. The former allows a more effective method of seeing a large dispersed client group. Every team member holds a small caseload, each of whom is seen for intensive therapy or specific ongoing work such as counselling. The majority of referrals, however, are treated in a more indirect manner through the active participation of the carers, social workers and any person in regular contact with the client. This enables other CMHT members to disseminate their skills amongst a wider group of people than would otherwise be possible using the more traditional methods.

Although based on a key worker system, other members of the CMHT do become involved with the client on a partnership basis during initial stages of assessment. This helps to achieve a global view of the client's strengths and weaknesses thus avoiding the danger of concentrating on one specific aspect whilst neglecting another. In addition there is the benefit of learning about the skills of other team members in a practical situation.

Basic principles

1.   It is important for the occupational therapist to look at the whole person who has a personality with special needs. He has to be taught, as far as possible, the skills which will assist him to be independent in daily living, socially acceptable, able to live with others and maintain a useful role in the community.
2.   It is essential to be familiar with a variety of approaches to treatment. For example, behavioural techniques are useful in teaching skills although the degree of sophistication is

adapted to suit individual clients.[6] The neurodevelopmental approach[7] is used to help those clients with cerebral palsy and allied disorders to maximise physical abilities, minimise the influence of abnormal reflexes and prevent further deformities.

3.   Therapy, by working towards objectives, is essential in helping the client, the therapist and others to know exactly what and how he is expected to do a task. It also helps in the process of evaluating the programme.

4.   Communication is vital between the occupational therapist, the client and others involved especially if confusion is to be avoided. Joint assessments and therapy programmes will show a united front.

Assessments

There are three types of assessments which can be undertaken depending on the needs of the client. First, to assess the general level of function. Second, specific assessments such as playing, and suitability for work (usually in the form of skills or task analysis before specific interventions are devised). Third, psychological testing if required.

The aims of the above assessments are:

(a)   establishing a baseline of the client's abilities;

(b)   identifying his needs;

(c)   deciding priorities for therapy and appropriate methods of therapy;

(d)   determining likely progression of therapy and ultimate goals and providing a measure of progress;

(e)   evaluation.

The following example describes such an assessment.

> A young woman who was employed by the local authority as a kitchen assistant in a day centre was referred by the personnel department following complaints about her work habits by the other staff. The main problems seemed to stem from her irregular attendance, poor personal hygiene, lack of initiative and slow pace of work which demanded constant supervision. At this stage she was transferred to another kitchen to obtain an unbiased assessment from a different staff group. They experienced similar problems which appeared to be compounded by the intense

pressure of work that occurred at peak times during the day. The local authoirty were relucant to give her notice and felt that an occupational therapy assessment would identify her strengths and the skills which she lacked in relation to work and, through this knowledge she could be redeployed to a more suitable post.

Using the Copewell work skills rating scale,[8] an assessment was carried out by observation of the client at work and interviewing her immediate supervisor. Her vocational interests and knowledge using the illustrated vocational inventory[9] were established; the results showed a limited understanding of the various elements of employment and an almost exclusive bias towards the caring professions. It was interesting to note that the client avoided the test material related to catering which gave rise to discussion about her attitude to her present job. It transpired that she disliked her work but was unable to initiate a change so had remained begrudgingly in her current position.

The final stage of assessment involved the client experiencing a variety of tasks in which she had expressed an interest. This also enabled the occupational therapist to observe her work skills in situations which the client enjoyed. Overall, she demonstrated a higher degree of initiative, concentration and accuracy of work than had been previously seen by her employers. Her speed of work remained slow and although she had difficulty in following instructions the assessment had clarified the method of teaching most appropriate to her needs.

From the recommendations made by the occupational therapist, the local authority were able to successfully transfer the client to a post in an old people's home which enabled her to maximise her skills in a less-pressurised environment. She is now a care assistant.

A selected range of assessment procedures and materials are available and are listed at the end of this chapter.

Therapy

Some of the prerequisites of physical abilities which need to be looked at have been covered in the chapter on the disabled child. Kiernan[10] has suggested four factors which need to be taken into account when planning a programme, particularly for those who are severely handicapped.

1.   *Rewards.*   Does the client have any likes which can be used as rewards in therapy or teaching sessions?

2.   *Educational blocks.* Has the person a behavioural problem or disability which hinders his learning? For those who are immobile, a programme can be devised to enable him to be placed in various positions. In other cases, such as self-mutilation, ways of eliminating the behaviour must first be considered and then a programme of activities planned to help his general development.

3.   *Socialisation and communication.* Does the person respond to others? Does he have a way of communicating his needs? If he is to develop he must first accept and like other people (it is interesting to note that those unable to communicate are not always seen as 'human' by the general public).

4.   *Reach and grasp.* Can the client reach and grasp for things? If this skill is not developed, the client will be unable to do many self help, play or work activities. Perkins, Taylor and Capie[11] added that any intensive therapy or teaching should focus on the following:

      (a) Can a client sit down at a table without any fuss?
      (b) Does he look at the person when his name is called?
      (c) Does he look at the object he is working with?
      (d) Does he co-operate – doing what you expect him to do if he understands what you want, and is capable of doing it?

Therapy may involve both individual and small group work.

Individual work

Advantages

1.   Undivided attention can be given to each, thus allowing him to concentrate on the activity with minimum distraction.

2.   It enables more time and concentration to be given to specific tasks.

3.   It is particularly useful for certain activities, such as teaching attention control, sensory and perceptual motor skills.

When undertaking all programmes it is important to keep up-to-date records (see Mary's activity chart below)

The following case study describes how the occupational therapist worked with a child and her parents at home.

The community team received a request from a teacher wanting someone to teach a family how to help their handicapped daughter. The team agreed that the occupational therapist should take the initial visit to Mary and her parents at home. Mary's family were caring and co-operative although they did not appear to appreciate that their daughter had a specific handicap. They talked about ways of helping Mary to become independent with self help and play skills. The parents and the occupational therapist subsequently visited the school where they saw Mary performing tasks not otherwise done at home such as feeding herself with a spoon. Consequently, she was encouraged to do so at home by improving her sitting position when she had her meals, borrowing the adapted spoon and plate from the school, and her mother holding her right hand. Through prompting by teachers and her mother, an improvement was gradually seen until Mary was able to use the spoon without any help. This took three weeks.

Meanwhile, Mary was given some play activities to do at home. Those activities which she did at school were first introduced which included posting circles into a box, taking a scarf off her face and unscrewing a rabbit in the barrel. These activities were recorded on an activity chart,[12] an example of which is shown in Fig. 21.

Once the parents began to feel confident with the progress being made they were then asked to keep a record of Mary's use of the toilet for a two-week period, i.e. Mary was to be taken to the toilet at the appropriate times. The result of this was that she began to use the toilet properly from time to time.

The family and the teacher received ongoing support from the occupational therapist and encouragement in maintaining the training programme and each was informed of Mary's progress at school and home.

Activity chart designed for Mary

Name: Mary

Activity: The game 'Peek-a-boo' – with a towel

Long term aim: To help Mary to be aware of people and to help her realise that things still exist when they disappear from sight.

Terminal objective: Mary will remove a towel from her face on request.

Criterion from success: Nine to ten times for three consecutive days.

Equipment: a large towel.

	Monday	Tuesday	Wednesday	Thursday	Friday
1.	⊘	⊘	⊘	✓	✓
2.	⊘	⊘	✓	✓	✓
3.	⊘	✓	✓	✓	✓
4.	✓	⊘	✓	✓	✓
5.	⊘	⊘	✓	✓	✓
6.	⊘	✓	✓	✓	✓
7.	⊘	⊘	✓	✓	✓
8.	✓	✓	✓	✓	✓
9.	⊘	⊘	✓	✓	✓
10.	✓	✓	✓	✓	✓

Date	Comments	Initials
17 February 1985	Criterion achieved; Mary will now take a towel from her mother's face	CSH

Fig. 21 An activity chart.

Procedure: Encourage Mary to sit on a chair facing you. Catch her attention, and then cover her head with the towel. Say 'take it off'. If she does, praise her and mark a tick on the chart. If she does not remove the towel repeat the request and hold her hand to remove the towel. Praise her and mark a circled tick on the chart. Repeat ten times per session.

Group work

Advantages
1.   It enables clients with similar needs to be seen together at the same time.
2.   It provides opportunities for interaction, social skills and learning skills such as taking turns and working together.
3.   It eases the pressure on clients.
4.   It enables a wider range of games and activities to be used.
5.   It enables the clients to practise and generalise skills taught on a one to one basis.

When planning group work, it is necessary to select those with similar needs and abilities, and devise a balanced programme of activities.

The following describes a group approach in which three mildly mentally handicapped men attended a closed social skills group.

> The group was run by the occupational therapist and clinical psychologist over a period of six weeks. All the men were experiencing a similar problem, namely, over-anxiety in social and/or unfamiliar situations. Their anxieties had grown to the extent that they avoided many events and experiences which had created a cramped and lonely lifestyle for them.
>
> Each session lasted two hours. It began and ended with relaxation with a break being taken midway. The first session was used to introduce the group members to each other, explain the purpose of the course and 'brain-storm' a list of stressful situations. These situations were then arranged according to degree of stress. Commencing in the first session with the least stressful situation and subsequently moving through such situation using role play, discussion and feedback as each task was covered. At the end of each session, the group members were given a task to be carried out during the following week to reinforce what was undertaken during the session.
>
> Both therapists had some doubts over the success of the group owing to the abstract nature of the situations identified, but these were quickly allayed as the group members gained confidence and became eager to correct each other during the role play.
>
> The outcome of the course resulted in one member finding employment after ten years of attending a day centre whilst the other two members presented a marked increase in self-confidence and esteem.

Other areas of practice

A large proportion of time can be spent in a variety of community settings such as day centres, employment training units, hostels and group homes. The success of an occupational therapist can be assessed not only by what she can achieve with the client but by how successfully other staff understand and carry out the prescribed training or therapy programme.

Involvement with training colleagues and education of the public on the needs of the mentally handicapped person is important and can be achieved through exhibitions, lectures and workshops.

Detailed discussions with his key worker, other members of the team, parents and carers of the reasons for the prescribed programme and the progress made will help educate all of the role of occupational therapy.

Planning new services

The occupational therapist should also be involved with the planning of new services, such as buildings for new units, and the development of extra services required. These may include day activities for those being transferred from long stay hospitals.

Acknowledgement. We would like to thank P. Ward, B.Ed. and S. Inglesfield B.A. (Hons) Dip COT for their constructive comments and help with this chapter.

References

1. G. E. Gathercole, *Residential Alternatives for Adults who are Mentally Handicapped*, British Institute of Mental Handicap, 1981.
2. J. Tizard, I. Sinclair and R. V. G. Clark (Eds), *Varieties of Residential Experience,* London: Routledge and Kegan Paul, 1975.
3. DHSS, *Better Services for the Mentally Handicapped*, London: HMSO, 1971.
4. Campaign for the Mentally Handicapped, *The Principles of Normalisation*, Campaign for the Mentally Handicapped, 1973.
5. G. B. Simon (Ed), *Local Services for Mentally Handicapped People*, British Institute of Mental Handicap, 1981.
6. W. Yule and J. Carr, *Behaviour Modification for the Mentally Handicapped*, London: Croom Helm, 1982.
7. K. Bobath, *A Neurophysiological Basis for the Treatment of Cerebral Palsy*, London Spastics International Medical/William Heinemann, 1980.
8. E. Whelan and H. Schlesinger, *Copewell Work Skills*, Copewell Publications, 1979.
9. E. Whelan and S. Reiter, *Illustrated Vocational Inventory*, Copewell Publications, 1980.
10. C. Kiernan, *Analysis of Programmes for Teaching*, Globe Education, 1981.
11. E. A. Perkins, P. D. Taylor and A. C. M. Capie, *Helping the Retarded – a systematic behavioural approach*, British Institute of Mental Handicap, 1983.

12. S. Bluma, M. Shearer, A. Froman and J. Hillard, *Portage Guide to Early Education*, National Foundation for Educational Research, 1976.

Further reading

S. Ayer and A. Alaszewski, *Community Care and The Mentally Handicapped,* London: Croom Helm, 1984.

M. Bayley, *Mental Handicap and Community Care*, London: Routledge & Kegan Paul, 1973.

M. Butts, D. Irving and C. Whitt, *From Principles to Practice*, Nuffield Provincial Hospitals Trust, 1981.

M. Copeland, L. Ford and N. Solon, *Occupational Therapy for Mentally Retarded Children*, University Park Press, 1976.

Department of Health & Social Security, *Helping Mentally Handicapped People in Hospital*, 1978.

C. H. Hallas, W. I. Frazer and R. C. MacGillaray, *The Care and Training of the Mentally Handicapped*, Wright PSG (7th edn), 1982.

E. F. Lederman, *Occupational Therapy in Mental Retardation*, Charles C. Thomas, 1984.

N. Malin, D. Race and G. Jones, *Services for the Mentally Handicapped in Britain*, London: Croom Helm, 1980.

G. B. Simon (Ed), *Modern Management of Mental Handicap – A Manual of Practice*, MTP Press, 1980.

D. Sines and J. Bicknell, *Caring for Mentally Handicapped People in the Community*, Harper & Row, 1985.

Useful addresses

Association of Professions for the Mentally Handicapped, 126 Albert Street, London NW1 7NF.

British Institute of Mental Handicap, Wolverhampton Road, Kidderminster, Worcestershire DY10 3PP.

British Epilepsy Association, Crowthorne House, New Wokingham Road, Wokingham, Berkshire, RG11 3AY.

The Campaign for Mentally Handicapped People, 16 Fitzroy Square, London W1P 5HQ

Kids & Kids, Bedford House, 35 Emerald Street, London WC1.

MENCAP – The Royal National Society for Mentally Handicapped Children and Adults, 123 Golden Lane, London EC1Y 0RT.

The Spastics Society, 12 Park Crescent, London W1N 4EQ.

A selected range of assessment and therapy materials

Assessment

J. Hogg and N. Rayne, *Assessments in Mental Handicap – A Guide to Test Battery & Checklist*, London: Croom Helm, 1986.

J. Jenkins, D. Felce, J. Mansell, F. Connie and D. Dell, *The Bereweeke Skill Teaching System*, NFER – Nelson Publishing Co., 1983.

P. Mittler (Ed), *The Psychological Assessment of Mental & Physical Handicaps*, London: Tavistock Publications, 1976.

E. G. Roach and N. C. Kephart, *The Purdue Perceptual Motor Survey*, Charles Emerrill, 1966.

G. B. Simon, *The Next Step on the Ladder: Assessment and Management of the Multi-Handicapped Child*, British Institute of Mental Handicap, 1981.

J. Whitehouse, *Mossford Assessment Chart for the Physically Handicapped*, NFER – Nelson Publishing Co., 1983.

C. Williams, *The STAR Profile: Social Training Achievement Record*, British Institute of Mental Handicap, 1982.

Test agencies

NFER (National Foundation for Education Research) – Nelson Publishing, Co., Darville House, 2 Oxford Road East, Windsor, Berkshire SL4 1DF.

Test Agency Limited, Cournswood House, North Dean, High Wycombe, Bucks.

Therapy materials

M. Bender and P. J. Valletutti, *Teaching the moderately and severely handicapped*, Vols I, II and III. University Park Press, 1976.

S. Bluma, M. Shearer, A. Froman, and J. Hillard, *Portage Guide to Early Education*, NFER – Nelson Publishing Co., 1976.

J. Comins, F. Hurford and J. Simms, *Activities and Ideas*, The Winslow Press, 1983.

E. Nicholls, and E. Mott, *Individual Learning Programme*. Royal National Society for Mentally Handicapped Children and Adults.

F. Mercer, *Activities Digest*, The Winslow Press, 1985.

S. Moule, L. William, and J. Holland, *Educational Rhythmics in Practice: starting and running a programme with the mentally handicapped*, BIMH, 1984.

Chapter 16

Ethnic groups

SHEILA EDEN
Occupational Therapist (paediatric and mental handicap services), Tower Hamlets, London

To discuss the diversity of cultures that exist in Britain today is impossible in a few pages and one person alone cannot possibly understand the numerous subtleties that exist in cultures other than the one they themselves come from. It is therefore not the intention within this chapter to discuss different cultures in any great depth but to share with readers some of the experiences gained from working amongst people with a different culture. It is hoped that by highlighting differences it will enable occupational therapists with little experience of different ethnic groups to become more aware of the impact different cultures have on our society.

Fashions come and go, and at the moment the term 'ethnic minority' is a fashionable term, being found in many official documents. An ethnic minority can be described as a group of individuals who consider themselves separate from the general population and who are seen by the community at large to be distinct because of one or more differences such as racial origin, skin colour, language, religious beliefs and practices, or dietary customs. Unfortunately, like many labels, its frequency of use produces abuse and to many the term 'ethnic minority' implies that the user is referring only to this country's black or Asian population. This should not be the case as any reference to ethnic minorities includes all cultures, black and white alike, that are different from that of the indigenous population.

Patterns of immigration.

It is inadvisable to consider multi-ethnic cultures without first looking at the patterns of migration that have occurred in this country. Having some knowledge of the reasons behind immigration to Britain does assist occupational therapists in becoming more aware of cultural differences.

Immigration to Britain is not a new phenomenon as this country has a long history of accepting, with varying degrees of tolerance, peaceful immigration from different parts of Europe. Jewish, Italian, Greek and Cypriot communities have become well established in various parts of Britain for many generations. Prior to the beginning of the Second World War this immigrant population was small and predominantly white. Immigration on a large scale started as a result of war and poor economic prospects in large parts of the Commonwealth.

Post-war Britain has become a multiracial society with about half the immigrants coming from Europe, the white Commonwealth and Ireland. The other half have come from the new Commonwealth countries of Asia, e.g. India, as well as Vietnam, China and Africa.

During the 1950s Britain was desperately short of unskilled labour for its economic revival, and so started to recruit overseas workers. Many prisoners of war also chose to remain in Britain bringing their families here to live. The influx of Poles, Hungarians, Ukrainians, Czechoslovaks, Italians and Jews brought changes and new traditions to the British way of life. This has meant that in most areas of Britain some aspect of the cultures of all these groups has been integrated into what we now regard as British culture.

By 1952, as a result of the McCarran–Walter Act, the United States closed its door to West Indians wishing to work in America and consequently many looked to Britain for employment. Large employers such as London Transport opened recruitment offices in the West Indies to assist prospective immigrants and for the next ten years West Indian immigration was at its peak.

In the next decade, during the 1960s, Asian immigration took place following the war which resulted because of political differences between India and Pakistan. This created the eventual partition of Kashmir, the Punjab and later Bangladesh. The loss of farms and poor prospects of jobs in their own countries made Asians look to Britain as a result of this unrest. At about the same time the

African nationalist movement caused severe economic and political pressures on the large Asian community in East Africa. Families were forced to leave as refugees, abandoning their extensive properties and businesses, and thus looking to Britain and India for safety.

Sociologists have described this process of migration in terms of a push and pull factor. The push factors are wars, religious persecution, political unrest and unemployment. The pull factors are good employment, prospects of a booming economy, good social and health services, political stability and peace. The process by which people come to Britain is important as it often influences the lifestyle which they adopt here.

The vast majority of the first immigrants to Britain were young men. Many were single, but others left families and dependants behind. Most were unskilled, illiterate in English and had little in the way of capital. West Indians had the advantage of knowing the language, though adjusting to the climate was difficult. Britain experienced full employment during this period and immigrants had little difficulty finding work although most were within the low pay sector of large industrial cities.

Like Britons abroad, they naturally grouped together in small communities according to their country of origin. Once settled they found homes and sent for their families. The subsequent influx of women and the birth of children have increased the size of these communities, leading to the appearance in some cities of a large minority whose skin colour makes them instantly recognisable as immigrants. Ironically more than half of these children have been born in Britain and most have never seen their parents' country of origin.

Britain has therefore in less than thirty years become a multiracial, multicoloured nation. For many of the first immigrants, such as Mediterranean Europeans, assimilation appears to have been superficially easier as their culture was similar to the indigenous population. It has been the increased number of immigrants from Asia that has perhaps presented British society with the most complex challenge. Although often grouped together by the native white Briton, the various ethnic groups are very different from each other, in language, dress, religion, family structure and diet. It is perhaps because the most recent arrivals to Britain are so different that the indigenous population is becoming more aware of the need to understand these differences.

Problems of adaptation

The arrival of immigrants into a community brings with it inevitable stresses during the initial period of adjustment. For therapists working with new immigrants it is important to remember that families may experience different levels of culture shock when coming to Britain. The severity of such a shock is related to the amount of change experienced and may be initiated by unsympathetic officials and exacerbated by difficulties in obtaining accommodation or employment. Adult members of a family can develop various changes in attitudes and behaviour which can cause children to become anxious and insecure. Fortunately most groups receive considerable support from the rest of their own community or from established family members.

At the moment few children are arriving as immigrants, apart from those who are joining fathers and other family members already established in Britain. These are mainly from Pakistan and Bangladesh. Children who can be instantly categorised as being 'non-European' because of skin colour or facial appearance may have great difficulty in establishing their true self and gaining acceptance and integration into the community as ₍ whole.

Communication

For many children, particularly the more recent immigrants, the first four years of their lives are spent speaking their mother tongue, usually with little contact with English except for the television. On reaching school age many children are unable to speak English, putting them at an instant disadvantage.

All ethnic groups basically learn two versions of English, colloquial English for the streets and standard English for school, alongside their own native tongue. Therapists should become aware of how information is disseminated within families. Most rely on children for interpretation and their abilities can be very variable. All information, whether verbal or written, must be presented in a form that can be easily understood and should not contain ambiguities.

Cultural differences

For many children the predominant problem is the conflict of values that exist at home and in the community, e.g. school. For many ethnic communities there is a distinct cultural difference between the expected roles of men and women. Older children, particularly teenagers, often feel caught between two cultures and have conflicts and difficulties in reconciling the two patterns of behaviour. For example, girls from Mediterranean or Asian communities may be expected to stay at home in the evenings and not join their peers in mixed social gatherings. This could cause a greater problem with integrating the young handicapped into social activities, e.g. PHAB or other groups. For some the prospect of an arranged marriage and the lack of freedom this can bring when compared with white British girls can be deeply disturbing.

It is helpful to have some idea of the reason, which is usually the same in each group, why a family came to Britain since this may influence their readiness to adapt to life in this country. Groups who maintain strong links with home by frequent visits and live in a close knit community with their own shops and organisations may not need to alter their lifestyle very much. Those who have been forced to leave their country because of political or religious persecution are more likely to accept the reality of permanent residence here. Since there is little prospect of returning home, British culture is more readily adopted.

Specific differences

Two areas that can produce the most anxiety amongst therapists are the use of correct titles and how to act in the home situation. It is for this reason that these two areas have been selected for particular comment.

Naming systems

For the majority of occupational therapists a referring letter is the first contact with a named client. For many ethnic groups the formal title used, e.g. Mr S. Cirpan, is similar to the British system and no difficulties arise. The naming system used in Britain however is not universal and the categories used, i.e. surname, christian or first name and middle name, can be meaningless to some ethnic groups. In Britain the first name is usually the one used by family and friends and the last name is always the family name or surname. These can be easily identified as the sequence of each name indicates its use.

Names originating in Asia and China, however, need a different approach. Asian names are confusing to a non Asian because they lack a common surname and cannot be matched to the British naming system in one easy procedure. For some Asian groups, such as Muslims, a further complication arises. Male and female members of the same family will have a different name for each other, making the identification of family members using the British system difficult. For example, Afia Begum's husband could be called Mohammed Ali Khan.

This creates numerous problems for the statutory authorities who invariably register the name of Begum as the surname and Afia as the first name. Further confusion occurs as children are given different names to their parents, with males often having honorary titles before or after their names. It is because of these differences that many people attending hospital may have more than one set of records. To attempt to remedy this problem the NHS training authority introduced a training pack in 1981.

In order for occupational therapists to simplify their own record keeping something similar to the following example is recommended.

> Client's name: Nasima Begum
> Father's name: Mohammed Ali
> Mother's name: Afia Khatun
> Family name: Khan
> Religion: Muslim

This way the father's name and his family name form an integral part of the child's name and it is then possible to identify members of the same family.

Another ethnic community that produces difficulties when trying to adapt names to the British system is the people of Chinese extraction. Here the surname usually appears at the beginning of a person's name, e.g. Mun Wy Ming. In this case Wy Ming is the first name, with the central part of the name, Wy, denoting the generation that person has come from. Some women within these communities do not change their surname on marrying but the children will take their father's name.

Families from many ethnic groups are now adapting their own naming system to fit the British style. Because this can lead to further confusion it is advisable that therapists ask the families for assistance when visiting and a clear explanation made in their records.

In the home

A successful visit (Photo. 9) can be achieved if the therapist uses a sensible and sensitive approach which should be essentially the same for all clients. From experience most professionals have little knowledge of different cultural, religious and dietary customs and thus the common difficulty experienced by therapists is the anxiety of not wishing to offend the family they are visiting. The most important fact to remember is that people are people irrespective of the cultural group to which they belong. Meeting people from a different ethnic background to one's own can produce feelings of inadequacy and awkwardness. The therapist should therefore be prepared to ask for assistance from the families themselves. If the therapist can acknowledge any cultural difference early in their relationship with the family, a more open approach will be possible. By employing this two-way process, trust and understanding can develop quite quickly and the true nature of problems can be identified.

The initial visit is important in establishing the right relationship with the client and family. The therapist should ensure that the correct introductions are made, a full explanation is given about the

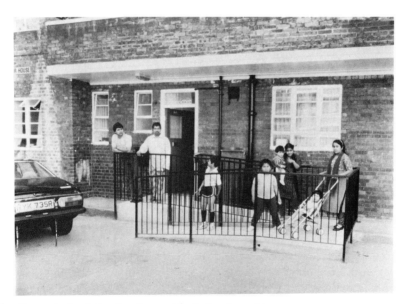

Photo. 9 An Asian family outside their adapted home.

reason for the visit and who has asked for it to take place. By completing these formal introductions any confusion over the purpose of the visit can thus be minimised. This will also assist in relieving anxieties that may be present for people with little experience of the British medical system. The right approach will produce positive attitudes towards receiving any future assistance.

One of the fundamental problems for all ethnic groups is the ability to understand and communicate with the various statutory authorities. Even for people born in Britain these services can appear confusing, as the amount in unclaimed benefits each year graphically illustrates. For ethnic groups unfamiliar with the complexities of the British health and social security system small problems can become major anxieties and so clear, accurate and concise information must be given.

Therapists should be careful not to fall into the trap of using the length of residency in this country as a barometer for assessing an individual's knowledge of the various statutory authorities. Knowledge of individual services is gained by the amount of contact families have with the various statutory bodies. This gives a better indication of whether people understand the functions of these departments than the amount of time an individual has been resident in this country.

Assessment

Like any assessment the therapist should first help with whatever the client and their family consider to be their greatest difficulty, leaving other problems to later. Although essential matters should be dealt with in this way some people will be unable to admit that they cannot perform certain functions, especially the more intimate activities such as managing the toilet unaided.

Even when a common line of communication has been established a therapist's greatest difficulty is in accurately interpreting the information given. A very important factor to bear in mind, which can cause confusion, is that the client will often offer information he thinks the therapist has come to hear, as would be their normal social practice, rather than what they really feel. This can cause a great deal of confusion unless rectified quickly. Some people will need an interpreter and may feel unable to communicate their private fears or anxieties via a known friend or family member, especially if this is a child. Therapists should be sensitive to these problems and arrange for an independent interpreter in such cases.

Before offering advice or equipment therapists should be aware that some of the solutions suggested, though sensible within one's culture, may be unacceptable to another. When visiting clients it is not uncommon for therapists to find a lack of response to previous advice given. If this occurs the therapist should not be discouraged but endeavour to discover the reasons behind such apparent lack of co-operation. By taking the initiative a therapist may discover that the client's initial response was not accurately interpreted.

The main aspect of any therapist's role is to develop and maintain the skills of independence. The way these skills develop will vary between cultures. This can be easily illustrated by looking at the skill of feeding which varies within different cultures in terms of cooking, eating and food habits. The British culture uses knives and forks, the Chinese chopsticks and many Asian countries use their right hand. If a handicap prevents a person from using their cultural eating method the obvious solution is not always the right answer. In Britain people are simply taught to use the hand most convenient irrespective of whether this means exchanging hands. For many Muslims simply transferring to their left hand for feeding is considered taboo as this hand is used for unpleasant tasks, e.g. managing the toilet.

Rehabilitation

The numerous communities within Britain have many cultural differences which can affect the way they live, eat and dress as well as affecting attitudes and values, e.g. towards women and children. Provided the foundations of mutal respect between client and therapist have been achieved then the barriers of communication can be considerably reduced.

Attitudes towards an individual family member's handicap can vary amongst all sectors of society. Many ethnic groups have very strong family ties with each member having a particular role to play. When a handicapped person is introduced into this environment, whether through birth, injury, or acquired, these traditions can often hinder that member's independence. In some situations status can change and this would be reflected in the person's ability to regain their previous family role. For example, a mother with poor mobility within the home could expect another female family member to take over her duties.

To many people, irrespective of their cultural group, the sharing of feelings within a group situation can be extremely difficult. For a number of ethnic minorities this public sharing of feelings is alien and becomes even more difficult if mixed sexes are also involved. Physical contact particularly in role play situations can also be unacceptable. Techniques such as meditation, or relaxation can be practised by some to an advanced degree. In certain situations these skills can be utilised for the benefit of all.

The intention here has been not to offer solutions to a number of difficulties that can arise when working with a multi-ethnic community but to emphasise the need for increased awareness amongst therapists involved with ethnic groups. Perhaps the key point to remember is 'sensitivity'. The therapist can never assume to know all there is to know, what she should do is open her mind to other viewpoints and remain willing to learn and appreciate cultural differences.

British culture will continue to undergo changes in the future and the external differences that exist today will gradually disappear. Therapists need to keep constantly in touch with these changes to enable fulfilment of their responsibilities to the community as a whole.

Further reading

Anil, Bhalla, Blakemore, *Elders of Minority Ethnic Groups*, 1981.

M. W. Arthurton, 'Some medical problems of Asian immigrant children', *Journal of Maternal and Child Health,* August 1977, pp. 316–21.

Healy Aslam, 'Present and future trends in the health care of British-Asian children', *Nursing Times,* August 1982.

V. Barnett, *A Jewish Family in Britain*, London: Pergamon Press, 1980.

J. Black, 'Child health in ethnic minorities – the difficulties of living in Britain', *Medical Practice,* Vol. 290, pp. 615–17, 1986.

P. Bridger, *A Hindu Family in Britain*, London: Pergamon Press, 1980.

W. Owen Cole, *A Sikh Family in Britain*, London: Pergamon Press, 1980.

Community Relations Commission, *Between two Cultures*, London: Commission for Racial Equality, 1976.

Shepherd Harrison, *A Muslim Family in Britain,* London: Pergamon Press, 1980.

'Asians in Hospital – What's in a Name', *Health and Social Service Journal,* July 1982.

Kings Fund Centre, *Ethnic minorities and Health Care in London*, London: Kings Fund Publications, 1982.

E. de H. Lobo, *Children of Immigrants in Britain, their health and social problems*, London: Hodder and Stoughton, 1978.

M. Pollack, *'Today's Three-Year Olds in London'*, London: Heinnemann Medical/Spastics International Medical Publications, 1973.

H. Tajfel, 'Social psychology of minorities' *Report No. 38, Minority Rights Group*.

Amrit, Wilson, *Finding a Voice – Asian Women in Britain*, London: Virago, 1978.

Useful addresses

Commission for Racial Equality, Elliot House, 10/12 Allington Street, London SW1 5EH.

Community Health Group for Ethnic Minorities, 28 Churchfield Road, London W3 6EB.

Ethnic Minorities Group, Middlesex House, 20 Vauxhall Bridge Road, London SW1.

Joint Council for the Welfare of Immigrants, 44 Theobalds Road, London WC1.

NHS Training Authority, St Bartholomews Court, 18 Christmas Street, Bristol BS1 5BT.

In addition to these most of the individual ethnic communities have their own national and local organisations who are always willing to assist with informal lectures and information.

Chapter 17

Employment opportunities

EILEEN E. BUMPHREY
Assisted by Hilary Schlesinger and Fenella Bemrose, Lambeth Accord, London

Despite high unemployment and early retirement, work is still important in the lives of most people. Not only is it important for providing an income on which to live, run the home and participate in leisure pursuits – but more importantly it is one of the major factors for the well being of the person and for providing social contacts. Unemployed disabled people lead a somewhat isolated life and are dependent on state benefits and pensions for their support. Life then becomes an existence rather than a worthwhile adventure.

Unemployment as assumed by society is a state that has been linked with poor physical and mental health for decades, and the benefit system and eligibility for services perpetuates this assumption. Various studies undertaken in many differing countries have shown that the consequences of unemployment lead to depression, low self-esteem, feelings of humiliation, of being superfluous, inferiority and worthlessness. Lack of confidence and a fear of failure are also deep problems for many. Society is now beginning to look on early retirement in a new way, as the opportunity for new pursuits, and doing those things that 'I have always wanted to do'. However, for the younger person the needs of work are still strong and it is unreasonable for them to be forced into a life of leisure and not have the right to acquire skills and qualifications with the ultimate aim of employment. The occupational therapist working with these people must be realistic about possible work opportunities within the surrounding neighbourhood, and only if absolutely necessary and desired by the disabled person himself should the therapist direct him into other worthwhile and meaningful pursuits.

Despite the fact that there is a record of disabled people in employment having an above average attendance and performing as well as any other employee, the legal quota of at least 3% registered disabled people in a workforce of twenty or more is very often not complied with. Why is it then that so many firms do not meet this requirement? Often it is that many of their current work force are already disabled in one way or another, but not registered as such. Also an employer, especially of a small firm, may never actually come into contact with disability and so he presents many apprehensions to the therapist when discussing a particular employee. Sometimes employers seeking disabled people do not get them applying for work and if they do, they often do not have the appropriate skills. On the other hand, it is quite common for disabled people not to know what skills they have, or what are appropriate jobs to apply for, as they often have not had the opportunity to explore these and gain qualifications and work experience.

Starting point

Before embarking on any rehabilitative programme with the ultimate aim of integrating a disabled person into employment, there are two things which the occupational therapist must do, as follows:

1. *Be well versed in what is available within the disabled person's local area,* in forms of Manpower Service Commission (MSC) employment incentive schemes, training, education and other resources such as sheltered work and community schemes. This includes MSC grants, aids and equipment available which change with great frequency and differ from area to area. Details of these can be obtained through the disablement resettlement officer and Job Centre.

2. *There are questions that the therapist should get the disabled people to ask themselves.* The occupational therapist must never make judgements about what they think a disabled person can or cannot do, and there should be no limit to expectations of the person and his potential within a degree of realism. As for anyone, an environment which gives a person space to think, and to adjust to possibilities

not thought of before, can induce self discovery and growth far beyond the expectations of the person himself and those working with him. The role of the therapist is to facilitate and aid the person in this self-discovery, with the specialist knowledge that they have, such as technology, aids, adaptations and resources that can open doors.

Local resources

Districts vary in the resources that are available but on the whole there will be a common pattern of types of service available. A range of provision from the public, private and voluntary sectors could well be used in providing opportunities for the preparation of work.

Community services

These include day centres, adult training centres (for the mentally handicapped), work centres, social education centres (SECs) and specialist community assessment teams for specific disability groups such as psychiatry, blind and deaf. Some of these services provide voluntary work opportunities such as helping others in a day centre which may be run by the local authority, social services or voluntary organisations.

These situations all have their advantages as well as their disadvantages. A work centre may provide opportunities for a form of employment and a small income, but these advantages could well be offset by the repetitive and boring nature of the work, with low expectations, unrealistic rewards given and the fact that the disabled person can only interact with another person in a similar situation. It does not provide an opportunity for integration. However, this may be better than sitting at home all day doing nothing, be a valuable starting point, and give future employers the knowledge of the ability acquired – e.g. specific skills, consistency in attendance. Job rehearsals can sometimes be arranged at these centres.

Employment services

The Manpower Service Commission through their DROs and disablement advisory services (these teams have a regional remit), provide help for the disabled especially with necessary aids, fares to work and adaptations to the employers premises. However, these are not available until a person is in employment. Special placement schemes are also often available, and other schemes encourage employers to seek disabled people. The therapist must be fully acquainted with all of these.

Some local councils have established opportunities for disabled people in an integrated setting particularly with training and business schemes. The occupational therapist will need to find out which directorate is responsible for these. For example, in Lambeth the employment promotion unit within the directorate of town planning holds all information about local resources which includes information about local industry, access and future planning of buildings.

Other possible local schemes

Pathway, run by MENCAP, is an employment and placement service for the mentally handicapped person and is one of many such schemes that are available. The chamber of commerce (the employers organisation), Rotary clubs and others are worth tapping to find out what is available in the local employment scene and who may be sympathetic employers to contact. A number of national organisations have local branches and involve themselves with the community in which they find themselves (e.g. Show Trust for special placement schemes). It is perhaps worth mentioning here that knowledge of local resources relevant for the employment of disabled people does not necessarily mean looking at special services or those schemes specifically designed for them. More and more the concept of integrating disabled people into the 'normal' provision of employment is becoming a definite policy.

Other contacts essential for inroads to work experience or employment

Many district councils and voluntary bodies have employment development officers/workers who will assist in this task. The majority of individual schemes have their own liaison worker who will advise on work experience placements, whereas other big employers have equal opportunity units such as district councils, British Rail, Shell and BP. Opportunities for disabled people apply in these just in the same way as all other members of the public.

Clubs and drop-in centres often require voluntary help to keep them going. Here, too, opportunities for gaining experience as well as socialising skills can be obtained.

Training

Many disabled people have minimal qualifications and therefore preparation for work may thus require returning to full time education preferably integrated into existing courses. Training opportunities vary throughout the country and again the therapist will need to know just what is available and where. Many local authorities have established their own schemes with, or independently of, educational establishments, whereas others are dependent on the MSC schemes and voluntary organisations.

MSC schemes

These include the following:
1.   The regional training office will provide information about what exists and what is planned for the future. Contact can also be made at the local council offices regarding current and future schemes available in the vicinity.
2.   Specialist employment advisers with a responsibility for advising and recruiting to training schemes are based in the job centres. These include YTS, TOPS, and other community programmes.
3.   College-based courses – information of these are available at local further education colleges and adult education institutes.

Education authorities

These authorities also play their part and the specialist careers officer can assist with many queries. They are based in the careers office of the central education department. Adult education and further education courses can often accommodate disabled people and the special needs co-ordinator will advise on their suitability. Not all courses are college based; some can be undertaken as correspondence or distance-learning courses.

Assessment

Employment rehabilitation is not different from the whole rehabilitation process – it is part of it. Consequently the assessment for employment rehabilitation should be much the same as that used for any other aspect of handicap or social disadvantage. Assessing and teaching work skills is important, but the occupational therapist must at the same time help to restore confidence, resilience and resourcefulness in order that the person can tolerate exposure to the demands of work.

Community-based assessment and work preparation needs the liaison with employers – either the handicapped person's present or future employer. Liaison will need to be with others who may be involved in the decision making such as disablement resettlement officers, specialist workers, such as those for the blind, and other professions such as clinical psychologists, physiotherapists and social workers.

In a few places around the country local vocational assessment teams (Asset Teams) are established to give basic assessment for local job opportunities, and trial periods within the work setting. Other areas have regionally based employment rehabilitation centres (ERCs) run by the MSC, where assessment, vocational guidance and work practice can be given. However, for the majority of community occupational therapists none of these facilities are available to them and consequently other resources have to be used.

Assessment should commence with the basic social skills such as use of public transport (if necessary), handling money, interaction with colleagues and personal care outside the home environment. The level of concentration and communication skills will also need to be considered with the possible help of other health professionals. Until confidence in these basic requirements is acquired, the success of the disabled person obtaining gainful employment is questionable.

Assessing a person's potential for work cannot be achieved without the full participation of that person. He or she must be committed to the exercise and really *want* to work. Unless the motivation is really quite high at the beginning then much time will be wasted. Motivation can be raised as the process progresses, but if it is not there at the beginning the disabled person will not be able to take the disappointments that may arise along the way, and consequently this may lead him into deeper despondency.

An accurate work assessment should increase the disabled person's knowledge of his own aptitudes and abilities as well as give a realistic understanding of his own skills. Assessment therefore starts with knowing what the person wants and allowing him to express his hopes and fears about employment. All people looking for work do so with a wide variety of expectations. Some may be wrongly seeking work as the answer to all their problems, or to avoid looking at more immediate issues, whilst others are realistic, knowing what they want, but do not have the knowledge or abilities to know how to go about it. An engineer looking for retraining in computers so that he can work from home following a diagnosis of multiple sclerosis has very different expectations from a teenager leaving college with learning difficulties. The occupational therapist should therefore be prompting the disabled person to ask himself such questions as:

'Do I feel ready for work?'

'What sort of work do I want to do?'

'What do I want from work – basic pay? Hours? Geographical area?'

'What are my marketable skills and qualifications? What can I offer an employer?'

'What am I doing to find work?'

'What difficulties do I have in finding work?'

'How can I overcome these difficulties?'

'What has been the effect of my disability on previous applications and jobs?'

'What are my family's expectations?'

'Will I be able to cope with the stresses and pressures imposed, meeting deadlines, working full time, making relationships, and dealing with conflicts?'

The answers to these questions must then be matched to the job opportunities, and a realistic understanding of what is available locally.

Return to a previous job may require a visit to the employer. A full understanding of what the work involves, awareness of the demands and pressures are necessary in order to support and prepare the employee for a return to work. Problems should be discussed and resolved at an early stage thus preventing long periods of frustration, possible redundancy, and loss of work habit. Special equipment may be required, such as an adaptation, aid or jig in order to succeed. Finance for these is available through the MSC. Apprehensions and misunderstandings on the part of the employer or colleagues may need to be fully discussed especially where there are psychiatric problems. Prejudice is often the result of fear through not knowing or understanding.

Liaison with social workers could also be necessary to establish basic pay incentives. For example, a disabled person receiving invalidity benefit and family allowances may have to earn a considerably high salary to make the incentive worthwhile. They may do better to look at alternatives to work and receive therapeutic earnings for voluntary work.

Assessment must essentially explore a person's abilities and match them to job requirements. There is no simple relationship between any particular job, the environment, attitudes, and actions of other people. So, for example, a solicitor who develops a hand tremor may find it has little effect on his work, whereas the dentist may have to abandon his career. A man with a manic personality may succeed as a door-to-door salesman, but would have disastrous consequences pursuing office work.

Much work has been done on evaluating the core skills necessary for work, which are transferable to a variety of work situations. Many different work assessment forms have been devised and are currently in use. However, the main aim for assessment must always be to give the disabled person the opportunity to evaluate his own strengths and weaknesses.

The following check list may be useful for those working in the community for the assessment of job analysis and task performance.

Work environment

Repetitive/varied	Dirty/clean
Isolated/with others	Noisy
Teamwork	Machinery
Pressurised	

Education

Qualifications	Functional writing
Functional reading	Functional maths

Sensory perception

Texture recognition	Colour discrimination
Position sense	Spatial perception
Temperature discrimination	

General work habits

Independent travel	Use of telephone
Attendance/time keeping	Social skills
Appearance and personal independence	

Physical abilities

Grip/Grasp	Hand-eye co-ordination
Finger dexterity	Posture
Manual dexterity	Mobility
Steady handiness	Lifting/Balance
Manipulative skills/speed	Sight/Hearing/Speech
Bi-manual co-ordination	

Work skills

Job adaptability	Expressive communication
Supervision	Emotional stability
Quality/accuracy	Concentration
Care and safety in use of equipment	Relationships with colleagues
Exercising foresight and initiative	Self confidence.

Preparation for work

Once the answers to all the above questions are known a plan of action can be devised together with the disabled person which could well include the following:

(a)   sorting out DHSS benefits by the social worker;
(b)   gaining the GP's opinion;
(c)   resolving problems with transport;
(d)   establishing what local opportunities are to be pursued.

Specific skills needed by the disabled person for applying effectively for jobs include the following:

1.   *Job search skills*
    (a) looking for and finding out about possible jobs;
    (b) visiting Job Centres;
    (c) writing initial letters to employers requesting application forms or enquiring about possible opportunities;
    (d) completion of application forms;
    (e) writing a CV;

(f) choice of referees and building up reliable ones (this can often be done after work experience is gained);

(g) use of telephone.

Videos to back up training in these areas are available from COIC and MSC.

2.   *Interview skills.* Confidence and a positive self image is important at interviews, without being over confident. It is important that they should also help to put the employer at ease about their disability and its effect on the proposed work situation.

As with any person applying for a job, the disabled person needs to learn how to sell himself. The use of video can be extremely valuable in a role play for an interview; for example, one young man stated 'I did not know my hair was as bad as that'! This method can also help to improve one's self image (see Appendix: Pre-work Course).

Work experience

Contacts with local employers are essential if inroads are to be made and opportunities for work experience and future employment. Employment liaison workers, whose sole job is to set up work experience placements for trainees on schemes such as YTS and equal opportunity units in larger firms who have a special interest in promoting the employment of minority groups will help with disabled people.

Work habits need to be developed or redeveloped. These should include:

(a)   work tolerance;

(b)   speed of activity;

(c)   timekeeping;

(d)   social skills;

(e)   travel.

These habits cannot only centre around the work environment, as the home must also be included, e.g., getting up in the morning, developing appropriate personal presentation, personal care and preparing lunch pack if needed.

Identifying core skills needed for work can be obtained through pre-work activities mentioned above. A check list could prove helpful in this and regular self-assessment.

General points to help disabled people prepare and seek for suitable work

A start should be made with jobs that are available locally, within easy travelling distance, and within the perceived expectations of employer and job seeker. This may initially have to be within a day/work centre, but the therapist should ensure that the disabled person does not get left there. Close monitoring is needed and regular reviews with the disabled person himself and centre staff should be established so that progress to the next stage can be made. Goal setting in these situations may be difficult owing to the lack of available opportunities within the locality.

Many disabled people want to work yet they find that employers only see their disabilities and not themselves as a person. They find it difficult to match their perceived abilities to those that the employer is looking for. Many employers want to employ disabled people and yet they think that if one has a handicap only simple sedentary work can be undertaken. Employers also find that some disabled people apply for tasks for which they lack the appropriate skills.

Somehow employer and employee need to be brought together.

By careful involvement, realistic assessment and successful placements, the occupational therapist can play an important role in helping employers to understand more fully the needs of disabled people and encouraging them to widen the range of opportunities open for them, as well as ensuring that the disabled person is aware of his real skills and has the confidence of applying them in a work situation.

Appendix – Pre-work course

The occupational therapist's role in work rehabilitation and assessment for people recovering from psychiatric illness does not only involve the identification of work potential; the development of the essential skills required to compete for employment on equal terms with other unemployed people is also of paramount importance.

The Manpower Services Commission defines long-term unemployment as 'unemployment of 6 months or more in those aged 18–24 years, and of 1 year or more in those aged 25 years or over'. The following course was designed for those not only disabled by a mental health problem, but for those whose job-seeking difficulties are further compounded by long-term unemployment.

The course aims to:
(a) help members become realistic about their preferences, experiences, capabilities and available job opportunities;
(b) provide information and advise on job-seeking methods and current employment practices;
(c) increase confidence, particularly in selling oneself to prospective employers;
(d) train in work-related social skills;
(e) provide a supportive environment for discussion of anxieties relating to employment thereby enabling members to acquire the necessary resilience and resourcefulness to cope with the demands of work.

Criteria for acceptance of referral. Before acceptance to the course, the occupational therapist will need to assess the proposed members suitability according to the following criteria, and in relation to their psychiatric condition.
1. Well motivated.
2. Have the potential ability to work, not only in relation to task performance but, more important, in terms of social skills.
3. Be prepared to make a commitment to the course – including assisting other members, actively participating and attending each session punctually.
4. Capable of seeking work on completion of the course.
There should be no age stipulations although an upper age limit of 40 years, depending on the individual, is realistic. The majority are likely to be within the 20–30 year age bracket.

Assessment

The effectiveness of the course for each member needs to be assessed by means of a *pre and post course inventory*. A self assessment measures factual knowledge before and after the course. It also identifies the ability to handle difficult work situations and establishes self confidence and anxiety levels. The inventory is compared with the opinion of the course tutors and the practical results in terms of job placement and social competence.

Course content

Weekly sessions for a closed group of six members are held over a six-week period. At the end of the course each member is reviewed individually and future needs established.

Session 1 – Looking for work. This includes methods of job seeking and the interpretation of advertisements. The need for a realistic and positive attitude is stressed repeatedly.

Session 2 – Applying for a job. This considers application methods. Throughout the course each member uses an imaginary vacancy applicable to themselves.

Session 3 and 4 – Interview techniques. The emphasis is on self-presentation, non-verbal communication and personal effectiveness.

Session 5 – Problems at work. This deals with appropriate behaviour in dealing with various work situations and relationships.

Session 6 – Employment rights (relating to both employer and employee). An explanation of relevant forms and related matters.

The format of each session involves group discussion, standard social skills training techniques, role play with video, home assignments and feedback.

Following such courses, which can be held at the local job centre, over half of the participants were working in open, sheltered or regular voluntary work one month after completing the course. Those that remained unemployed continued to actively seek work. For the first time in two years one member was successful in getting interviews and obtained a temporary job which led to a permanent one. Of the three whose psychiatric state relapsed, one eventually progressed to sheltered work and another to voluntary work.

Besides tangible results, the secondary benefits of improved social competence are equally valuable, although more difficult to measure. Perhaps the comments of two members, but typical of others, are self-explanatory: 'I had become introverted since my illness and the course has brought me out'. And another who said, 'I have learnt to explain my condition in both words and writing which has given me confidence, and already that has proved a success'.

Acknowledgements. Our thanks go to Liz Flood for her contribution to the Pre-work course and for sharing her work carried out in the local job centre where the course is held.

Further reading

M. Greaves and B. Massie, *Work and Disability 1977*. Disabled Living Foundation, 1978.

Richard Groves and Francis Gladstone, *Disabled people – a right to work?* NCVO Policy Analysis Unit, Bedford Square Press, 1981.

Hobson and Mays, *The Theory and Practice of Vocational Guidance*. London: Pergamon Press, 1968.

B. Hopson and M. Scally, *Build your Own Rainbow – a work book for career and life management*. Leeds: Lifeskills Associates, 1984.

M. Kettle, *Disabled People and their Employment: a review of research into the performance of disabled people at work*. Association of Disabled Professionals, 1979.

Code of Good Practice on the employment of Disabled People. Manpower Services Commission.

Occupational Therapy Reference Book. British Association of Occupational Therapy, 1986.

Useful information

Careers Occupational Information Centre, MSC Sheffield. Bibliography and list of videos available on career-related subjects.

Manpower Services. Pamphlets and publicity on employment rehabilitation provision. Available from MSC, Moorfoot, Sheffield.

Careers Research and Advisory Centre (CRAC) provide a variety of courses to assist teachers and students (14–18+) with preparation for work. CRAC Publications, Hobsons Ltd, Bateman Street, Cambridge CB2 1LZ.

Chapter 18

Leisure pursuits

PHYLLIS WESTERN

Leisure is an important ingredient in everyone's life and is becoming more so as the retirement age creeps down and more people than ever live to old age. The modern scourge of unemployment also leaves many people with many spare hours to fill and so the subject of leisure is very topical. Positive ways of coping with leisure time are therefore important. Physical activities such as keep fit and medau are much discussed as being vital for maintaining health and well being. This applies for the disabled person just as much as the able bodied especially as spare time can pose deeper problems. The obvious practical problems relating to leisure pursuits and to activity centres, such as access and the need for some practical help from the able-bodied sector, are additional factors that need to be considered.

Attitudes toward leisure depend on the person's personality and the family expectations; they can be partly inherited such as the skills of a craftsman, or be acquired. The chosen pursuit is usually closely related to personal idiosyncrasies and may be deeply satisfying through the opportunity for expressing a person's inner self.

Constructive use of leisure time for all, whether elderly, mentally handicapped or physically disabled, is vitally important as it can make all the difference between thoroughly enjoying a full and positive life, or merely existing. Having something positive to think about, and aim for, is not only a wonderful ego booster, but it is important for relaxation, a balance to life, and to raise the handicapped person's self esteem.

Leisure activities therefore that promote positive thinking and some constructive achievement, however small this may be, will help the disabled person to realise his full potential. Boosting self confidence will not only create a whole person, but will also help him to feel that he can take his place in society and contribute something to it. Development of a strong character is a great asset to any disabled person, and participation with able-bodied competitors will contribute to this development. One who is shy and retiring is doubly handicapped. The disabled child or adult will need to learn to project his personality beyond his particular handicap so that he will appear to others as a person in his own right, who just happens to be disabled.

For the more handicapped person, leisure time and activities play an important part in their lives. In some instances it can be a substitute for work and provide an opportunity of participating in a creative activity; of being introduced to wider horizons of interest; increasing social contact; satisfy a competitive nature; and help to compensate for the lack of employment opportunities and its related status.

For those who have become suddenly disabled through trauma or an acute illness leisure pursuits can

(a)   help during the initial period of readjustment from fitness to handicap thus helping the person to re-orientate himself and accept a very different lifestyle;

(b)   compensate for the frustration which sudden deprivation of fitness brings;

(c)   provide an essential means for regaining self-esteem, achievement and social contacts;

(d)   provide a worthwhile alternative to work.

Previous training and interests will naturally influence the activities chosen and many will succeed in these with help. However, the resultant handicap may in fact create a deeper frustration in the realisation that he is unable to succeed in it as well as he could. The occupational therapist therefore needs to encourage the disabled person to explore other fun situations so as to discover unknown and untapped abilities.

For those disabled people of a higher intellectual bracket, sedentary academic activities will be all absorbing. However, attendance at adult education classes can pose problems for them although the interaction provided by these classes may compensate for all the difficulties.

Total rehabilitation includes leisure and thus the therapist must be ready to help each person discover an appropriate interest in which he can actively participate and make a contribution, even if it is only keeping a score card. Within an institution group discussions led by a therapist are a well-known means for stimulating interests. These can easily continue within the community, for example, by encouraging participants of a group to relate to the others details of a certain TV or radio programme. These groups can be held in each others homes if suitable. This approach can be a useful first step but encouragement to wean them away from the group into an existing 'class' organised by the local amenities department or education centre will enable further progress in rehabilitation.

Leisure possibilities must be considered in the context of the following:

1. The local vicinity and the facilities that are available within it.
2. The individual's level of education and previous occupation.
3. The individual's temperament – whether he is a sociable or solitary person.
4. Previous participation and interests.
5. Home conditions
6. Family and friends willing to help.
7. Financial implications – e.g. subscriptions, cost of outlay for equipment.
8. Fatigue level and physical comfort.

When embarking on a new hobby there will be many barriers to overcome such as transport, architectural features at the place of activity, and toiletry arrangements.

Clubs and societies

Like most people, the disabled person enjoys being a member of one or more of the local clubs, societies and associations and it is a good way for them to make new friends and broaden their horizons. The sense of being accepted, belonging and being part of any group, is essential to being secure; this acceptance must however be on the same terms as the other participants. This will mean that they will have to make the effort to enrol, to attend regularly and to mix with new people. Once this is achieved they will be able to reach their full potential.

Although joining a club provides opportunities for social activities which the disabled person might not otherwise have, they also provide opportunities for them to contribute to the group. This is important and a point which is often overlooked, for the more disabled a person is, the more they have to 'take', and disabled people often long for the chance to 'give'.

There are clubs solely for disabled people such as the St Raphael Clubs, which can be found in most towns. Some disabled people find comfort in being with others like themselves and discovering that they are not alone with their problems. However, others long to be integrated with their able-bodied friends. Such clubs, as PHAB (physically handicapped and able-bodied) clubs are for both and actively attempt to integrate the physically handicapped and able bodied which can be very rewarding for everyone concerned.

There are also a great number of groups centred around specific interests such as gardening clubs or amateur radio societies. These are of course open to all and it may take more effort and courage for the disabled person to enrol into one of them. However, as well as meeting other people with the same interest, the ratio of able-bodied members will be much higher, thus promising plenty of practical help to overcome any practical difficulties encountered. As disabled people join in these societies and clubs the more they will be understood and accepted into society.

Getting started

As a general rule the disabled person needs a lot of practical help and encouragement to get started with a leisure activity. Occupational therapists can help enormously by providing this help, encouragement and continued support. They should also be prepared to make realistic suggestions of possible activities that are practical, achievable and acceptable to the person concerned. It is important not to over-estimate the energy and capabilities of handicapped people because this will only lead to frustration and disappointment. It can be very disheartening for them to discover that they cannot, after all, quite achieve something that they had dared to hope for. Disabled people get used to failure and disappointment, and consequently will often tackle something new with a rather pessimistic attitude. Extra effort on the part of the therapist therefore is needed in order to kindle a spark of interest in something new.

Suggested activities

The range of possible activities is limitless, and of course the choice will depend upon the individual. Most disabled people wish to live their lives as normally as possible and so it follows that they would rather participate in those leisure activities arranged for all if at all possible. Even so, these must be realistic.

I have a personal tale to tell which I feel is relevant here. I am in a wheelchair and have no arm movement. Once I was persuaded to take part in a game of darts! The dartboard was placed flat on the floor in front of me, and someone lifted my arm as necessary with me clutching the dart in my hand. At the appropriate moment, as my arm was pivoted through the air, I had to let go of the dart and maybe it would land on the board! No treble twenties, needless to say, but the important point is that I gained no satisfaction whatsoever from this exercise, it bore no resemblance to actually playing darts and illustrates that one can go too far in trying to achieve normality.

For some, evening classes and other forms of further education are an answer; but a disabled person may need help with finding out what is available and when, enrolling, and maybe with transport. It is no use finding the ideal course when the person has no means of transport, access to the premises is difficult or courses held in an evening when energy may well already be spent. There are so many everyday pursuits in which they can become involved, such as fishing, gardening, amateur radio, handicrafts, painting, flower arranging and writing, to name but a few.

Gadgets and adapted equipment may be needed and can be used to great advantage. Even the simplest aid, used with a little ingenuity, can mean that a handicapped person can manage to join in with some activity which he could not otherwise manage. For example, mobile arm supports, when correctly fitted and balanced, will often facilitate enough movement in weak arms to enable that person taking part in several games and hobbies, which need only a small amount of arm movement. Strategically placed stands, pads and remote control switches all have their place. For example, a severely disabled person can take up photography using an automatic camera

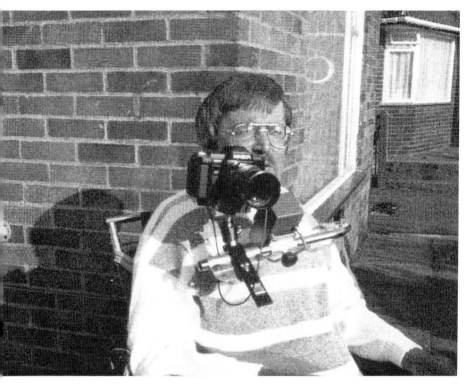

Photo. 10 A specially adapted camera.

screwed onto a stand held at eye level and with a simple remote control switch attached which the photographer can manage himself (see Photo. 10).

Sports

All sports can be enjoyed by disabled people, whether as participant or observer. Some will achieve seemingly impossible feats by sheer determination to compete and do well. For example, some handicapped people do great things in the world of athletics as is seen regularly in the Disabled Olympics and other national sports events where amputees take part in both high jumping and long jumping very successfully. Others pride themselves in being excellent score keepers.

Water is a medium which can facilitate easier movement, and consequently many elderly and disabled people enjoy swimming. Sailing is a developing sport for handicapped people as sailing clubs are introducing facilities for disabled people. Consequently many are now enjoying this invigorating sport. A square rigged sailing ship, the *Lord Nelson*, has just been launched which is designed specifically to enable disabled people to handle the sailing themselves. Ramps, hoists, special tracks on deck to prevent wheelchairs rolling about, and a special compass which will enable blind people to steer have been installed for this purpose. The Peter Le Marchant Trust also provides holidays afloat for disabled people and their families.

Other outdoor pursuits are all very healthy and should be encouraged. Horse riding is popular and, like swimming, is an activity in which disabled people can compete on a more equal footing with their able-bodied counterparts. Archery is another similar example.

Gardening is a very versatile activity because it can take place both indoors and outside, alone, and in groups. Tending houseplants and growing small things in pots can be very satisfying. In the garden, the appropriate planning of ramps, paths and raised flower beds can mean that people with all kinds of disabilities, including wheelchair users, can enjoy gardening for much of the year. Many tools with special grips and long handles have been designed with the disabled and elderly person in mind. A very comprehensive and useful book to refer to on this subject is the Leisure and Gardening section of Equipment for the Disabled.

Finally reading is enjoyed by many. Large print books are available for the elderly and partially sighted person. Books are also recorded onto cassettes for blind and partially sighted people and those who cannot physically manage to read books. Most local libraries have these and some have 'talking newspapers'.

Many leisure activities and hobbies can take place at home and these too should be encouraged especially for the housebound or for those winter days when it would be detrimental to go out. Active participation in any form of absorbing activity whether reading, needlecraft, modelmaking or painting that brings achievement enhances positive thinking and relationships.

There must be something to suit almost everyone – the choice stretches as far as the imagination goes and the therapist should act as an enabler.

Holidays

Everyone needs a break occasionally whether it be a weekend spent a few miles from home or a week abroad, and disabled people are no exception. Holidays are also important for their carers whether they be family, friends or employees, for without them relationships between all concerned become strained and create many unnecessary and unintentional problems. Handicapped people are more likely to become tense, bored and totally inflexible without a change of scenery and routine. A holiday will also often bring about a positive gain in confidence as well as physical well being.

Disabled people should be encouraged to participate as fully as possible in the planning and preparations of these as the challenge and anticipation can bring an enormous amount of fun and motivation as well as being very gratifying in itself.

Many will not embark on holidays because financially they are unable to meet the costs involved. Whilst many charitable bodies organise holidays for their particular group, these are not always the right type of break or holiday that is required. Social service departments and some charities however will help with financing a holiday, especially when a break for the carers is indicated. Some organisations arrange very interesting holidays and weekend breaks where able-bodied participants are on hand to help push a wheelchair over rugged terrain and other situations.

The type of holiday decided upon will largely depend on the physical abilities of the disabled person concerned, the feasibility of mode of travel, and accessibility of the chosen venue. Disabled people should not be afraid of being adventurous, including visits abroad, as much more is now possible and even the quite severely handicapped person can enjoy a wide variety of holidays both at home and abroad.

The right *accommodation* will need to be sought to suit the particular needs of the disabled person concerned by careful selection of brochures. Many hotels will happily accommodate disabled people (coded in AA, RAC and many other guides) and it is not always necessary to book into places which cater specially for them. However, accessibility and positioning of beds, electric plugs, bath, toilet and such like will need to be checked out well beforehand. In fact thorough detective work and early planning are good keywords. Many offering accommodation can often be very helpful when they know all the circumstances.

On the other hand some disabled people prefer to go camping and caravanning. Several sites both in this country and abroad are suitably equipped.

As well as the right accommodation, it is important to investigate carefully the local amenities. Many holiday resorts now have useful guides for the disabled visitor.

Travel arrangements must be carefully worked out well in advance. Air, rail and sea travel are becoming very aware and equipped for the disabled and elderly traveller and are introducing extra facilities and amenities to meet these needs. Full enquiries need to be made well in advance to let the authorities know exactly what the requirements are so that adequate preparation can be made, such as escorted wheelchairs in airports, seat reservations in central aisles, and opportunities for the elderly and disabled person to be seated in the aircraft before others are allowed on to the plane. Wheelchair users wishing to use a cross channel ferry need to check the size of the ship's lift as these can be very small.

Much encouragement and support is needed on a first journey away from the security of the familiar environment and a change from the usual tried and trusted routine can bring about many apprehensions.

My first tentative holiday since the onset of my disability was a week with a very trusted friend in a very ordinary little guest house in Bournemouth. I remember causing quite a stir as my friend made endless journeys carrying wheelchairs and various pieces of equipment, including a large respirator! Fortunately we soon made friends with the proprietors and other guests so much so that we had a marvellous holiday. To most people this would have been a very ordinary holiday but to me it was a tremendous achievement and gave me the courage and confidence to adventure further, including some exciting visits abroad.

Further reading

Ann Darnbrough and Derek Kinrade, *Directory for Disabled People*, Cambridge: Woodhead-Faulkner, in association with RADAR, 1986.

Equipment for the Disabled, fifth edition, *Leisure and Gardening*, Oxford Health Authority, Nuffield Orthopaedic Centre, Oxford OX3 7LD.

Holidays for the Physically Handicapped, The Royal Association for Disability and Rehabilitation. Available from libraries.

Further information

Leisure

British Association for Sporting and Recreation Activities of the Blind, 11 Ovolo Road, Stoneycroft, Liverpool 13. Tel: 051–220 2516.

Disabled Information and Advice Line (Dial), Central office, Dial UK, Dial House, 117 High Street, Claycross, Chesterfield, Derbyshire.

Disabled Drivers Motoring Club, 1A Dudley Gardens, Ealing, London W13 9LU.

The Disabled Living Foundation, 380–384 Harrow Road, London W9 2HU. Advice and comprehensive information on leisure.

National Clubs for Physically Handicapped and Able-Bodied (PHAB), Tavistock House, Tavistock Square, London, WC1H 9HY.

Holidays

AA and RAC Guides for holidays for disabled people available from AA and RAC centres and leading bookshops.

Disabled Living Foundation (address as above).

PHAB (address as above).

The Scout Holiday Homes Trust, Baden-Powell House, Queen's Gate, London SW7 5JS. Tel: 01-584 7030.

Summer Academy, Study Holidays at British Universities, Summer Academy, School of Continuing Education, The University, Kent CT2 7N.

Threshold Travel, Worldwide holidays for disabled people, Threshold Travel, Wrendal House, 2 Whitworth Street, West Manchester M15 W.

The United States welcomes handicapped visitors. Booklet available from USTTA, 22 Sackville Street, London W1X 2EA.

Useful addresses

Northern Ireland Council for the Handicapped (NIHC), 2 Annadale Avenue, Belfast BT7 3JH. Tel. 0232 640011. A federal member of the Northern Ireland Council of Social Service, provides a forum for voluntary organisations concerned with the disabled and their carers.

Wales Council for the Disabled, Caerbragdy Industrial Estate, Bedwas Road, Caerphilly, Mid-Glamorgan, CF8 3SL. Tel. 0222 887325. Co-ordinating organisation for voluntary groups in Wales. Information service on disablement issues, campaigns for better facilities for disabled people.

Scottish Council on Disability, 5 Shandwick Place, Edinburgh, EH2 4RG. Tel. 031-229 8632. The council provides a means of consultation between statutory and voluntary organisations for disabled people in Scotland. It also operates an information service.

Rehabilitation Engineering Movement Advisory Panels (REMAP), 25 Mortimer Street, London W1N 8AB. Tel. 01-637 5400. Through its 92 panels (branches) in the UK, REMAP provides an engineering solution to problems of disabled people when no aid already on the market is a satisfactory answer.

Association of Visually Handicapped Office Workers (AVHOW), 14 Verulam House, Hammersmith Grove, London W6. Tel. 01-749 1372. AVHOW is concerned with blind and partially sighted people in office employment and aims to improve their prospects of promotion.

The Royal Association in Aid of the Deaf and Dumb (RADD), 27 Old Oak Road, Acton, London W3 7HN. Tel. 01-743 6187. RADD aims to meet the spiritual, social and special needs of people of all ages who have a hearing impairment from birth or childhood and so have needed a special education.

Royal National Institute for the Blind (RNIB), 224 Great Portland Street, London W1N 6AA. Tel. 01-388 1266. The RNIB works for the better education, rehabilitation, training and general welfare of all Britain's blind people.

Cruse, the National Organisation for the Widowed and their Children, Cruse House, 126 Sheen Road, Richmond, Surrey TW9 1UR. Tel. 01-940 4818.

Relevant legislation

Mental Health Act 1983

The Mental Health (Amendment) Act 1982 received the Royal Assent on 28 October 1982 making substantial amendments to the Mental Health Act 1959. However, all of the amendments are consolidated into the Mental Health Act 1983, which came into effect on 30 September 1983 and is now the only Act in force in the field of mental health. This legislation includes:

1. Setting up the Mental Health Commission to protect the interest of detained patients.
2. New requirements regarding the treatment of detained patients.
3. Procedures for the admission to hospital.
4. Mental health review tribunal procedures.
5. The term 'mental impairment' replaces 'subnormality'.
6. Introduction of formal 'approval' of social workers in mental health.
7. New powers for Courts to remand to hospital for reports or treatment and to require from regional health authorities details of what hospital places are available.
8. From 1 April 1983, informal patients in mental hospitals have been able to make a declaration which allows their names to be included in the electoral register.
9. Removes sexual deviation and dependence on drink or drugs as definable within the terms of mental disorder.

Education Act 1981

This Act relates to special educational needs and establishes a new framework for the education of children requiring special education provision whether in special or ordinary schools.

Section 1 of the Act gives effects to the recommendation of the Warnock Committee that the 1944 Act system of special educational treatment for pupils suffering from a disability of mind or body, who were formally classified in specified categories of handicap, should be replaced by special educational provision based on the special educational needs of individual children.

Section 2 amends existing duties and introduces new ones to accommodate the new and wider framework of special education. It also establishes the principle that all children in need of special education are to be educated in ordinary schools, so far as is reasonably practicable, and are to associate in the activities of the school with other children. This principle is subject to account having been taken of the views of the parents and, amongst other things, the ability of the school to meet the child's special educational needs.

For detailed information, see: DES Circular 8/81, 'Education Act 1981', and DES 1/83 (HC(83)3) (LAC1.)2), 'Assessments and Statements of Special Educational Needs'.

National Assistance Act 1948 (as amended by Local Government Act 1972)

Section 29 is of particular importance to occupational therapists as it is under this section that local authorities are given powers to promote the welfare of handicapped persons. The definition of 'disabled person' is persons who are blind, deaf or dumb, and other persons who are substantially and permanently handicapped by illness, injury or congenital deformity or such other disabilities as may be prescribed by the Minister. This continues to be the definitive definition for registration required in subsequent Acts, e.g. Rating (Disabled Persons) Act 1978 and the Housing Act 1974. The arrangements which authorities may make include:

1. Advice on available services.
2. Instruction in methods of overcoming the effects of disabilities.

3.   Provision of workshops and hostels for handicapped workers, home work and assistance in disposing of such produce.
4.   Provision of recreational facilities.
5.   Maintenance of registers of handicapped persons.

Section 30 enables local authorities to use and fund certain voluntary organisations providing these services act as their agents.

Sections 21 and 27 covers provision of residential accommodation.

Chronically Sick and Disabled Persons Act 1970

Section I requires local authorities to inform themselves of the number and needs of disabled persons (as defined in Section 29 of the National Assistance Act), to publish information on the services they provide under Section 29, to ensure that any disabled person using a service is informed of any other services which in the opinion of the authority is relevant to his needs.

Section II. Many of the formerly permissive functions of Local Authorities become mandatory, and the 'arrangements' which can be made to promote the welfare of the individual are translated into identifiable services. The Act requires that where a local authority, having powers under Section 29 of the National Assistance Act, is satisfied that in order to meet the needs of a disabled person ordinarily resident in their area, it must make arrangements for any or all of the services set out in Section II and is then duty bound to provide them under the general guidance of the Secretary of State. Hence the level of provision made in any authority will depend upon its definition of need.

The services to be provided are:

1.   Practical assistance in the home.
2.   Provision or assistance in providing radio, television, library or similar recreational facilities.
3.   Provision of lectures, games, outings or other recreational facilities outside the home or assistance in taking advantage of educational facilities that are available.
4.   Provision of, or assistance in, travelling to take part in these or other similar activities.
5.   Assistance in obtaining housing adaptations or additional facilities.

Disabled Persons (Employment) Act 1944

Section I defined 'disabled person' for employment purposes as one 'who on account of injury, disease (including a physical or mental condition arising from imperfect development of any organ) or congenital deformity, is substantially handicapped in obtaining or keeping employment, or in undertaking work on his own account of a kind which, apart from that injury, disease or deformity, would be suited to his age, experience and qualifications'.

The main provisions of the Act are:

1. The setting up of a 'Register' of disabled persons (maintained by the Department of Employment), the aim being 'to secure that the fact that a person's name is on the Register will afford reasonable assurance of his being a person capable of entering into and keeping employment, or of undertaking work on his own account'.

2. The provision of vocational training and industrial rehabilitation courses and establishment of industrial rehabilitation units now known as Skills Centres.

3. Introduced the Quota scheme whereby an employer who normally has, or even temporarily has, a workforce of 20 or more must, subject to certain exceptions, employ a quota of registered disabled persons (currently 3%).

4. Allowing the Secretary of State for Employment to designate certain categories of employment for registered disabled persons. (Only car park attendants and electric lift opertors are designated at present and this provision is rarely used in practice.)

5. Enables the Secretary of State to provide special facilities for the employment of seriously disabled persons.

Rating (Disabled Persons) Act 1978 (does not apply in Northern Ireland)

This Act enables rating authorities in England and Wales to grant rebate in respect of the rates chargeable on special facilities in a property required for meeting the needs of a resident disabled person.

The special facilities prescribed are:

1. A room predominantly used by and required for meeting the

needs of the disabled resident (whether for providing therapy or for other purposes).

2. Additional bathroom or toilet.
3. Central heating installation in two or more rooms.
4. Any other required facility.
5. Sufficient floor space for wheelchair use.
6. Garage, carport or land used (other than temporarily) for accommodating a vehicle required for meeting the needs of a disabled person.

All facilities have to be deemed to be required for meeting the needs of the disabled resident, i.e. 'are of essential or of major importance to his well-being by reason of the nature and extent of his disability'.

Disabled Persons Act 1981

Section I re *roadworks* amends the Highways Act 1980 and Roads (Scotland) Act 1970 to require local and highway authorities to have regard to the needs and safety of disabled and blind people when undertaking roadworks, and when considering providing ramps between carriageways and footways and to ensure that holes in the pavement or street are properly protected.

Section II re *orange badges*. Amends Road Traffic Regulations Act 1967 to increase penalties for the misuse of orange badges.

Section III re *public buildings*. The Town and Country Planning Act 1971 is amended to lay a duty on local planning authorities when granting planning permission to draw attention to the relevant sections of the CS & DP Act 1970 and the Code of Practice for Access for the Disabled to Buildings BS 5810: 1979. This duty applies to public buildings, offices, shops, railways and factories. In the instance of university and educational premises, the duty is to draw attention to sections 7 and 8 of the CS & DP Act and Design Note 18 'Access for the Physically Disabled to Educational Buildings'.

Section IV re *toilets for the disabled*. The Local Government (Miscellaneous Provisions) Act 1976 is amended to lay a duty to draw the attention of those providing lavatories at places of entertainment to the needs of disabled people, Section 6(1) and 7 of the CS & DP Act and BS 5810: 1979.

Section V re *directional signs*. This section replaces Section 7 of the CS & DP Act and requires those making provisions required by sections 4, 5, 6 and 8 and 8a to provide signs indicating facilities for disabled people and the appropriate route to those facilities.

Section VI re *provision of buildings*. In all sections of the CS & DP Act which impose a duty to pay regard to the needs of disabled people in the provision of buildings. This means provision in accordance with BS 5810: 1979 or, for educational buildings, Design Note 18, unless the developer can demonstrate to a 'prescribed body' that it is not practicable or reasonable to make such provision in that particular circumstance. This section applies to sections 4(1), 5(1), 6(1) and 8A(1) of the CS & DP Act and applies to England and Wales only. (There is a similar provision in sections 36 and 37 of the Local Government (Miscellaneous Provisions) (Scotland) Act 1981.)

Section VII re *access to buildings*. A new section 8B is inserted in the CS & DP Act requiring the Secretary of State to report to Parliament on his proposals for improving access for disabled people to public buildings and lavatories.

The Social Security and Housing Benefits Act 1982

This Act makes provision for a new scheme, housing benefit, to give help with rent and rates. Housing benefit brings together the two former schemes – supplementary benefit payments for rent and rates and local authority rent and rate rebates and rent allowances.

For further information see DHSS Circular HB(82)2, 'The Housing Benefit Scheme: Implementation'.

Public Sector Housing Act 1957

Section 91 requires housing authorities to consider housing conditions and needs of their district and that they have regard to the special needs of disabled people is made explicit in Section 3 of the Chronically Sick and Disabled Persons Act. Section 2 of the Act also gives Social Service Authorities the statutory power to assist with housing adaptation in both public and private sector housing.

Private Sector Housing

Housing Act 1974 Section 56 (as amended by Housing Rents and Subsidies Act 1974). This Act enables discretionary improvement grants to be made specifically for works required for making a dwelling suitable for the accommodation, welfare or employment of a disabled occupant, providing the dwelling is, or will become, his only or main residence.

It also enables mandatory intermediate grants to be made for installing standard amenities (WC, fixed bath or shower, etc.) or the installation of suitable alternative facilities where existing amenities are inaccessible to the disabled person.

Housing Act 1980

This Act is concerned with the standards governing the award of improvement and intermediate grants; of special significance for tenants and low-income owners. It also:

(a)   widens the scope of the repairs grants to deal with structural disrepair in old houses;

(b)   removes the rateable value limit in respect of improvement grants for work required for a disabled occupant;

(c)   enables secure tenants in the public sector and regulated tenants in the private sector to apply for improvement, intermediate and repairs grants.

For information regarding relevant *DOE circulars* – see Chapter 9.

Index

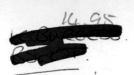